To Malinda

INTRODUCTION

One of the goals of the *Journal of Fire and Flammability* is to so guide its content that within five years a complete collection of issues would be the basic literature source in this field of technology. Compilations of Journal articles in areas of specific interest thus become a valuable literature resource, and the Fire and Flammability series of books embodies this concept.

Flame spread may be defined as the rate of travel of a flame front under given conditions of burning. This characteristic provides a measure of fire hazard, in that surface flame spread can transmit fire to more flammable materials in the vicinity and thus enlarge a conflagration, even though the transmitting material itself contributes little fuel to the fire. Because of its demonstrated relevance to life safety, surface flame spread, until recently, received most of the attention given to flammability characteristics.

The ten articles in this volume were selected from the *Journal of Fire and Flammability* because they represent the most up-to-date information available on surface flame spread.

CONTENTS

PAGE

The Mechanism of Flame Spread,
by R. S. Magee and R. F. McAlevy 1

Flame Spread Rates of Solid Combustibles in Compressed and
Oxygen-Enriched Atmospheres, by A. Nakakuki 28

Fire Studies in Oxygen-Enriched Atmospheres, by V. A. Dorr 35

Thermal Analysis of Combustion of Fabric in Oxygen-Enriched
Atmospheres, by A. M. Stoll and M. A. Chianta 51

Flame Spread Model for Cellulosic Materials,
by W. J. Parker 67

Quenching Distance for a Combustible Solid in the
Oxygen-Enriched Atmosphere, by K. Komamiya 83

Application of a Flame-Spread Model to the Oxygen
Index Test, by J. M. Funt and J. H. Magill 93

A Four-Foot Tunnel Test Apparatus for Measuring Surface
Flame Spread, by C. J. Hilado and P. E. Burgess 104

A Schlieren System for Fire Spread Studies,
by C. P. Butler 114

Quantitative Analysis of Prescribed Burning,
by P. J. Pagni 126

PUBLISHER'S NOTE

The Mechanism of Flame Spread

Richard S. Magee and Robert F. McAlevy, III

Combustion Laboratory
Stevens Institute of Technology
Hoboken, New Jersey

(Received June 7, 1971)

ABSTRACT

A number of factors influence flame spread rate, some in a way that results in large data scatter. The data reported in this paper were obtained using smooth-surfaced specimens with inhibited edges of reasonable scale in either vertically downward or horizontal propagating flames. Since the structure of the flame zone has never been studied, hypothesized models cannot be compared with any existing experimental evidence. As such, an impasse now exists which can be broken only if new studies concerning flame zone structure are made.

INTRODUCTION

The propagation of a flame over the surface of a combustible solid is an extremely complex process. In spite of the large body of experimental data obtained over the past six years, there still exists uncertainty as to which parameters exert dominant effects. However, since heat must travel from the flame to the unignited material, clearly, certain heat transfer modes must be involved. The motion of the gas at the leading edge of the flame is of potential importance. The gas-phase chemistry including oxidant concentration, inert diluent and pressure, as well as inter-diffusion of reactants, must also be considered. Finally, the influence of solid phase surface chemistry, thermal properties and geometry cannot be ignored.

In order to obtain some perspective on the relative importance of the various parameters on the flame spread phenomena, it is beneficial to examine the results from some idealized experiments conducted in five laboratories on flame spread under various conditions. The data to be examined were obtained in studies at Stevens Institute of Technology [1-4], Atlantic Research Corporation [5-6], Naval Research Laboratory [7], Linde Division of Union Carbide [8], and the U.S. Forest Service [9] since 1965. Much of these data are tabulated in a recent review paper by Friedman [10]. The tables which follow show data selected from these references which illustrate certain trends, and form the basis for speculation concerning the relative importance of the various parameters on the flame spread rate. Following

1

Table 1. Effect of Surface Roughness and Exposed Edges on Flame Spread Rate.

HORIZONTAL FLAME SPREAD

(a) Smooth polymethylmethacrylate, edges inhibited: 0.28 cm/sec
     Smooth polymethylmethacrylate, edges exposed: 1.2 cm/sec
     (STEVENS, O_2 at 1 atm)

(b) Smooth plastics, edges inhibited: 0.1 − 0.2 cm/sec
     Smooth plastics, edges exposed: 0.5 − 0.9 cm/sec
     Foamed plastics: 32 cm/sec
     (ARC, O_2 at 5 psia)

(c) Filter paper (LINDE)   0.36 cm/sec
     Smooth cellulose acetate (ARC)   0.03 cm/sec
     (air, 1 atm, edges exposed)

VERTICAL (DOWNWARD) FLAME SPREAD

(a) Smooth polymethylmethacrylate, edges inhibited: 0.33 cm/sec
     Smooth polymethymethacrylate, edges exposed: 1.96 cm/sec
     (STEVENS, O_2 at 1 atm)

Table 2. Effect of Sample Orientation on Flame Spread.

(a) Polymethylmethacrylate (edges inhibited)
     (STEVENS, O_2 at 1 atm)

     horizontal   0.28 cm/sec
     vertical downward   0.33 cm/sec
     vertical upward   rapid, erratic

(b) Cellulose acetate sheet (edges inhibited)
     (ARC, O_2 at 5 psia)

     horizontal   0.12 − 0.14 cm/sec
     vertical downward   0.12 − 0.15 cm/sec
     vertical upward   rapid, erratic

(c) Filter paper (edges exposed)
     (LINDE, air)

	1 atm	10 atm
horizontal	0.36 cm/sec	0.48 cm/sec
22.5°upward	0.63 cm/sec	1.35 cm/sec
45°upward	1.12 cm/sec	2.92 cm/sec
75°upward	2.92 cm/sec	4.20 cm/sec
vertical upward	4.6-7.4 cm/sec	5.9-8.1 cm/sec

Friedman these data are reported in metric units. (In contrast, the figures shown later are from recent publications by the authors, and these data are presented in English units.)

The effect of the physical nature of the combustible polymer on the flame spread rate is shown in Table 1. These results are for horizontal flame propagation on the upward-facing surface and vertical flame propagation down one side only. All data are for "still" environments — i.e. no wind. This table shows that a flame propagates approximately five times faster over a smooth surface when the edges are exposed than when they are inhibited. In addition, exposing the edges increases data scatter. Also the rough texture of the foamed plastic results in a two-orders of magnitude increase in propagation rate over that exhibited by smooth plastics with inhibited edges. This influence of surface roughness is also shown in Table 1, where filter paper, with a rough texture, is compared to smooth cellulose acetate. Even though these materials are chemically similar, the flame propagation rate over the filter paper is twelve times faster than over the smooth plastic. Thus, surface roughness and condition of the specimen edge powerfully influence the flame spread rate.

Table 2 shows the effect of specimen orientation on flame spread in a quiescent environment. The results for both polymethylmethacrylate and cellulose acetate indicate that there is little difference between horizontal flame spread rate and vertical downward flame spread rate. However, upward flame spread rate is much more rapid and erratic and very difficult to measure quantitatively. The Linde results with strips of filter paper indicate that the flame spread rate increases with the angle of upward orientation. (Their results also became quite erratic when the sample was 90° vertical and the authors suggested that, at the maximum, a 45° upward orientation be employed for reproducible results.) Also the flame spread rate increases by an order of magnitude from the horizontal to vertical orientation. Thus, it is concluded that specimen orientation also exerts a powerful influence on the flame spread rate.

Table 3 shows the effect of material chemical composition on the flame propagation rate. For the conditions stated, teflon would not propagate a flame once ignited,

*Table 3. Effect of Chemical Composition on Horizontal Flame Spread Rate. ***

(a)   Pure O_2, 5 psia (edges inhibited):

teflon (STEVENS)	0.00 cm/sec
polyvinyl chloride (ARC)	0.04 cm/sec
delrin (STEVENS)	0.04 cm/sec
nylon (STEVENS)	0.05 cm/sec
polyethylene (ARC)	0.11 cm/sec
cellulose acetate (STEVENS)	0.13 cm/sec
cellulose acetate (ARC)	0.14 cm/sec
polymethylmethacrylate (STEVENS)	0.14 cm/sec
polystyrene (STEVENS)	0.16 cm/sec
polypropylene (ARC)	0.18 cm/sec
"Tygon" — plasticized (ARC)	0.53 cm/sec

*Specimen width varied from laboratory to laboratory. Stevens employed specimens 3/8 in. wide, while ARC tested specimens 1/2 in. wide.

while Tygon, probably due to the great volatility of the plasticizer, propagates a flame the fastest. The remaining eight polymers seem to divide into two groups, polyvinyl chloride, delrin and nylon forming one group with a flame spread rate around 0.04 cm/sec; the other five, polyethylene, cellulose acetate, polymethyl-methacrylate, polystyrene and polypropylene having flame spread rates near 0.15 cm/sec. Thus, as one might expect, fuel chemistry influences flame spread rate. But only as much as other factors.

Table 4 shows the effect of specimen geometry on the flame spread rate. In (a) the data indicate a strong effect of the width of the paper strip on flame spread rate. In fact, the flame spread rate seems to be proportional to the width. However, the data in group (b) show somewhat different trends. In the case of horizontal flame spread, the flame spreading velocity increases by about 25% when the width is increased from 1.0cm to 5.0cm. On the other hand, for vertical downward flame spread over identical specimens there is no width effect. However, when a similar experiment was performed with a cellulosic material, (c), increasing the width from 2.5cm to 7.5cm resulted in a 30% increase in flame spreading velocity. Finally the data in group (d) indicates an opposite effect. Here for vertical downward flame spread, the flame propagates faster down a small rod than down a large rod. Hence,

Table 4. Effect of Sample Geometry on Flame Spread Rate.

EFFECT OF WIDTH

			vertical downward	horizontal
(a)	Paper strips (45°upward burning) (LINDE, in air)			
	0.6 cm width	1.8 cm/sec		
	0.8 cm width	2.4 cm/sec		
	1.2 cm width	3.1 cm/sec		
(b)	Polymethylmethacrylate* (STEVENS, O_2 at 1 atm)			
	1.0 cm width		0.33 cm/sec	0.28 cm/sec
	5.0 cm width		0.33 cm/sec	0.36 cm/sec
(c)	"Index" cards (vertical downward)* (STEVENS, air at 1 atm)			
	2.5 cm width		0.10 cm/sec	
	7.6 cm width		0.13 cm/sec	
(d)	Cellulose acetate (vertical downward) (ARC, O_2 at 5 psia)			
	1/8" diam. rod		0.37 cm/sec	
	1" diam. rod		0.23 cm/sec	

*edges inhibited

no general conclusion can be drawn concerning the influence of specimen scale in the direction parallel to the flame front on flame spread rate.

Table 5 illustrates the effect of environmental pressure on the flame spread rate in quiescent O_2/N_2 environments. The data in group (a), for horizontal flame propagation, show that for six polymers the pressure exponent is near 0.8, while for wood and paper the exponent is much lower, approximately 0.1. Friedman [10] suggested that this difference might be due to the presence or absence of edges, or it might be due to the different physical or chemical nature of wood or paper compared with the smooth polymers. However, more likely it is a consequence of the different behavior of thermally "thick" and thermally "thin" specimens. (Note: The concept of thermally "thick" and "thin" specimens, insofar as the flame spreading phenomenon is concerned, will be discussed in detail in the "Theory" section.) This is shown by the data in group (b). In this study, specimens of two different thicknesses were tested. As the results show, the "thick" specimens exhibited a very strong pressure dependence, while the "thin" specimens did not. Thus, the effective thermal thickness of

Table 5. Effect of Pressure on Flame Spread Rate in O_2/N_2 Environments.

$$V_\alpha \, P^\Phi$$

Material	Laboratory	Pressure Range (atm)	Oxygen Range (mole fr.)	Φ
(a) HORIZONTAL				
Polystyrene*	STEVENS	0.3–28	.46–1	0.76
Polymethylmethacrylate*	STEVENS	0.3–28	.46–1	0.82
Delrin*	STEVENS	0.5–15	1	0.80
Cellulose acetate*	STEVENS	0.3–28	1	0.72
Nylon*	STEVENS	0.5–15	1	0.75
Teflon*	STEVENS	4.4–28	1	1.10
Paper	ARC	0.5–1	.46	0
Wood				
Paper	LINDE	1–10	.21	0.12
Paper	NRL	1–5	.21–.31	0.13
(b) VERTICAL DOWNWARD				
Paper (thin)*	STEVENS	.3–28	.21–1	0.06
Paper (thick)*	STEVENS	.3–28	.21–1	0.63
(c) 45°UPWARD				
Paper	LINDE	1–10	.21–.5	0.46
Paper	LINDE	.2–1	1	0.38

*edges inhibited

5

the specimen has a strong influence on the flame spread rate. Finally, the data in group (c) indicate that the pressure exponent for 45° upward flame spread over paper is considerably higher than for horizontal propagation over the same material. This suggests a different mechanism may enter in this case, possibly reflecting the influence of free convective velocity. Thus, fuel bed depth as well as orientation can influence powerfully the flame spreading phenomenon, as demonstrated by the way they influence the pressure dependence of flame spread rate.

Table 6 shows the effect of oxygen content on the flame spread rate. In most cases nitrogen was employed as the diluent. However, the ARC data includes some runs with argon and helium as the diluent also. The propagation rates, with one exception, vary with a power of oxygen mole fraction either about 1.0 or somewhat greater than 2.0. It can be shown (see Theory section) that those specimens which exhibited exponents greater than 2.0 are in fact thermally "thick", while those with exponents near 1.0 are thermally "thin". Again, it is demonstrated that specimen effective thermal thickness strongly influences the flame spreading phenomenon.

Substitution of helium or argon for nitrogen changes the gas phase thermo-dynamic (e.g. specific heat) and transport (e.g. thermal and mass diffusivity) properties. Experimentally, the dependence of flame spread rate on inert diluent has been found to be strong [1, 10]. But the actual mechanism can be examined only through hypothesized models and their predicted results (see Theory section).

Flame spread rates have been found to be independent of fuel bed depth for depths greater than 0.1 in. or so [4, 19]. But they are inversely proportional to

Table 6. Effect of Oxygen Mole Fraction on Flame Spread Rate.

$$V \propto Y_{ox}^{m\Phi}$$

Material		Laboratory	Pressure Range (atm)	Oxygen Range (mole fr.)	$m\Phi$
(a)	HORIZONTAL				
	Polystyrene*	STEVENS	0.3–28	.46–1	2.3
	Polymethylmethacrylate*	STEVENS	0.3–28	.46–1	2.5
	Paper	NRL	1–5	.21–.31	1.6
	Paper	ARC	.3–1	.21–1	.96
	Painted surface	ARC	.3–1	.21–1	.91
	Foam cushion	ARC	.3–1	.21–1	2.06
(b)	VERTICAL DOWNWARD				
	Paper (thin)*	STEVENS	0.3–28	.21–1	0.90
	Paper (thick)*	STEVENS	0.3–28	.21–1	2.1

* edges inhibited

thickness for thinner sheets [3, 6, 10, 19]. This effect is rationalized in the Theory section using the concept of effective thermal thickness of the specimens. And as noted above, this effective thermal thickness exerts a powerful influence on the flame spreading phenomenon.

Flame spread rate increases with increasing specimen initial temperature [2, 21]. This influence is rationalized in the Theory section also. However, the parameter is very rarely varied in laboratory experiments.

The influence of "wind", or forced convective motion in the environment, on flame spreading velocity has been recently studied. Rothermel and Anderson [9] investigated the influence of low-speed convective motion (0-10 fps) in the direction of flame propagation on the flame spread rate over a bed of pine needles; and concluded that, for the flow velocities tested, the flame spreading rate increased exponentially with flow velocity. In another series of experiments conducted at Stevens, [2], tests were performed with forced convective motion (0.6-30 fps) opposed to the direction of flame propagation over two polymeric fuels. Both fuels exhibited increasing flame spread rates with increasing flow velocities until a "critical" flow velocity was reached. Further increases in flow velocity beyond this value resulted in a decrease in flame spreading velocity. It is concluded that wind velocity strongly influences the flame spread rate, although the nature of the influence is probably complex.

In summary, it is clear that a number of factors influence flame spread rate, some of them in a way that results in large data scatter in the laboratory experiments reviewed. To produce data that might be used to test theoretical predictions it is necessary to eschew experiments that involve specimens with uninhibited edges or vertically upward propagation; in fact, it appears that only horizontal or vertically downward propagation can be rationalized at present.

Specimen scale and roughness exert influence on flame spread rate, and these must be considered in experimental design. Since there is no way at present to specifically account for roughness effects theoretically, only data from "smooth" surface specimens are capable of rationalization. The specimen size normal to the direction of flame propagation should be sufficiently great to insure one-dimensionality of the phenomenon (as only one-dimensional theories have been published), but it is not clear how this can be established experimentally (e.g., see Table 4) at this time. And as a corollary, it is not clear how to "correct" for scale when comparing results from experiments that differ in this regard.

By using smooth-surfaced specimens with inhibited edges of "reasonable" scale in either vertically downward or horizontal propagating flames, a number of investigators have attempted to establish correlations between flame spreading velocity and the other variables cited above. Much of these data are reproduced herein. In the Theory section the more successful attempts to rationalize these correlations are reviewed. The hypothesized models differ mainly on assumptions concerning the structure of the spreading flame and the mode of heat transfer selected as being important. The next section is intended to show that there is no experimental basis for making these assumptions.

R. S. Magee and R. F. McAlevy, III

OBSERVATIONS OF THE FLAME IN LABORATORY FLAME SPREADING EXPERIMENTS

The Luminous Flame

During flame spreading, a luminous flame is observed moving along the specimen surface. The velocity at which the flame propagates is measured and reported as the flame spreading velocity — the dependent variable.

Generally speaking, the luminous flame rises from just above the fuel bed surface at some angle in the direction of propagation. At greater distances from the surface, the angle relaxes and the flame rises vertically upward. Parker [14] has recorded some of his observations of flame shape for vertical downward propagation and Wrubel [15] made similar observations for horizontal propagation. Sufficient observations have not been made to date to allow any general statement to be made concerning the influence of pressure and oxygen concentration, for example, on luminous flame shape. However, Wrubel's photographs indicate that luminosity increases as these parameters increase.

Lastrina [16] has observed that the luminous flame is blown back by an opposing wind and blown forward by a following wind. Perhaps the much greater data scatter associated with the latter case reflects the uneven heating exposure of the surface in front of the actual flame location by the "tail" that is blown forward, touching down here and there. At the very high wind velocities, characteristic of those produced in a solid rocket motor during the flame spreading phase of the ignition transient, Most and Summerfield [17] report that the flame spreading appears to be controlled by random heating to ignition of "hot spots" along the propellant surface.

Generally, in quiescent experiments the luminous flame exhibits a blue leading edge (representative of fuel-lean combustion) which becomes yellow (representative of fuel-rich combustion) at the back side, as it moves along the fuel bed [6, 13, 14 and 16].

To the authors' knowledge, there have been no studies of the aerodynamics associated with flame spreading, nor have there been any measurements of temperature distributions or gas composition through the flame in the gas phase. In short, the structure of the propagating gas phase flame has never been investigated.

Temperature Distribution on the Fuel Surface Beneath the Spreading Flame

Extensive measurements of the temperature distribution have been made for polymethylmethacrylate in various oxygen-inert diluent environments [18]. Surface-mounted, fine-wire thermocouples were employed. It was found that the surface temperature rose continuously from its initial value to a final value in a very small distance, — between 0.15 cm and 0.40 cm depending on environmental conditions. And that the final temperature (approximately 400 C) was independent of conditions.

Bhat [21] employed the same technique with cellulosic specimens at atmospheric conditions and also found that the distance for temperature rise was very small, although data scatter was much greater — probably due to difficulty in mounting the thermocouples.

In addition, to these data, Parker presented the results of an experiment with a cellulosic material that indicated a preheat distance of 0.15 cm [14].

Thus, the flame region is very limited in extent.

Heat Flux in the Flame Region

To the authors' knowledge, there have been no measurements of heat flux through the gas phase in the flame region. So it is impossible to discern the relative importance of conductive, convective and radiative heat transfer. However, as will be seen in the Theory section, this is an important assumption in the various flame spread models. But without data for support, these assumptions are pure speculation.

The surface temperature distributions have been employed as a basis of calculating heat flux normal to and parallel to the solid surface at both surface and subsurface locations [16]. The heat flux normal to the surface is in all cases greater by an order of magnitude than the heat flux parallel to the surface (i.e, in the direction of propagation).

REVIEW OF MAJOR FLAME SPREAD THEORIES

Recent theoretical investigations by Magee, McAlevy and Lastrina [1, 2], de Ris [11] and Tarifa, Notario and Torralbo [13] represent the most advanced attempts to date to describe the process of flame spread over a combustible material in an oxidizing atmosphere. Each investigation considered an idealized flame spread problem for which a simplified model was formulated and analyzed. In References 1, 2, and 11, the authors produced simple algebraic expressions that correlate the flame spreading velocity and appropriate parameters.

All assume that flame propagation is a continuous process whereby heat, released by chemical reaction, is transferred in some fashion to the unburnt fuel bed surface. This causes the fuel bed surface temperature to increase, increasing the fuel pyrolysis rate and hence the production of gaseous fuel molecules. These molecules then enter, by diffusion and convection, the chemical reaction zone where their combination with oxidizer molecules liberates the heat necessary to continue the flame propagation process. This overall view suggests the phenomenon called flame spreading is composed of a number of individual, but coupled, phenomena (e.g. chemical reaction, heat transfer, pyrolysis, etc.). Mathematical description of all these processes results in a set of coupled linear and non-linear partial differential equations whose exact solution is presently impossible. Thus, simplifying assumptions are made which hopefully do not destroy the essential features of the problem, but reduce its mathematical description to a level that yields to analysis. The ability to correlate empirical data is typically taken as justification for the simplifying assumptions employed.

This section will review the physical processes considered in each investigation as well as the major assumptions employed. In addition, the resulting flame spread expressions are presented. The reader is referred to the individual publications for the details.

Magee, McAlevy and Lastrina [1, 2]

Extensive, well-defined experiments by Magee and McAlevy [1] in quiescent O_2/inert environments have shown that the flame spreading velocity (V) over thick horizontal polymeric fuel beds is a strong function of environmental pressure level (P) and oxygen mole fraction (Y_{ox}). All of the data could be correlated by a universal power-law relationship of the form $V \propto (PY_{ox}^m)^\Phi$. They found that the surface temperature increased from its initial value, T_o, to a maximum surface temperature, the fuel "burning temperature", T_b, in a very small distance, δ. (For polymethylmethacrylate, PMM, the burning temperature was equal to 750 F independent of the gas-phase environmental conditions and δ varied from 0.06 in. to 0.15 in. depending on the gas-phase environmental conditions) [1]. Following the steep temperature rise, the surface temperature was found to remain constant at T_b. They postulated that V is controlled by the processes taking place within the small distance δ, the "ignition region" at the leading edge of the spreading flame adjacent to the surface. A continuous, diffusive gas-phase ignition model of the flame spreading phenomenon was postulated and a simplified analysis of this model, supplemented by experimentally-determined surface temperature profiles in the ignition region, yielded the same power-law relationship as that exhibited experimentally [1]. It was concluded that gas-phase processes in the ignition region strongly influence the flame spreading phenomenon. The solid phase was not considered explicitly, so its influence on the phenomenon could not be assessed.

In a more recent investigation [2], Lastrina, Magee and McAlevy developed theoretical flame spread expressions capable of explaining the influence of both gas and solid-phase parameters on the flame propagation rate. To accomplish this, they postulated, as they had in Reference 1, that the processes controlling the flame spreading phenomenon occur in the very small ignition region at the leading edge of the spreading flame adjacent to the surface, and attention was focused on this small region. The solid phase energy equation was uncoupled from the gas-phase conservation equations and solved separately, retaining as a boundary condition the heat flux into the surface from the adjacent gas phase. Their solid and gas-phase analysis are outlined below.

Solid Phase Energy Equation:

Two different approaches are used to obtain solutions to the solid-phase energy equation: an unsteady one-dimensional heat conduction approach (based on the assumption that heat conducted parallel to the fuel bed surface is negligible compared to heat conducted normal to the fuel bed surface), and a control-volume approach (based on the assumption of negligible heat conduction across the interior boundaries of the control volume). These approaches yield analytical solutions which differ only by a numerical coefficient for the flame velocity over thin and thick fuel

10

beds in terms of the physically important parameters.

The time required to heat the surface from T_o to T_b, the ignition period, is the time for the flame to propagate the distance δ, i.e. δ/V, where V is the flame spreading velocity. For the unsteady, one-dimensional heat conduction approach two cases were investigated: one for a constant surface heat flux during the ignition period; and the second, for a linearly increasing surface heat flux with time during the ignition period. The control volume approach employed assumed surface temperature distributions as boundary conditions. These approaches yielded:

Thermally Thin Fuel Bed $\qquad\qquad (\bar{\tau}<1.0)$

$$\dot{Q}_s = \rho_s C_s V' \, \tau' \, (T_b - T_o) \qquad\qquad (1)$$

Thermally Thick Fuel Bed

$$(\tau>1.0)$$

$$\dot{Q}_s \cong 0.8 \, (K_s \rho_s C_s \delta V)^{\frac{1}{2}} (T_b - T_o) \qquad\qquad (2)$$

where V' is the thin fuel bed flame spreading velocity (as opposed to the symbol V used for the thick fuel bed flame spreading velocity), $\dot{Q}_s$ is the total heat flux into the solid fuel bed, K_s, ρ_s and C_s are the thermal conductivity, the density and the specific heat of the solid respectively, τ' is the thin fuel bed thickness and

$$\bar{\tau} = \tau (K_s \delta / \rho_s C_s V)^{\frac{1}{2}} \qquad\qquad (3)$$

is the dimensionless fuel bed thickness. Hence a natural criterion, $\bar{\tau} \approx 1.0$, evolves from the analysis, which defines the critical thickness separating thermally thin from thermally thick fuel bed behavior insofar as flame spreading characteristics are concerned.

Gas Phase Conservation Equations:

As stated previously, any general attempt to describe mathematically the gas-phase results in non-linear partial differential equations. This obstacle is circumvented by the authors by avoiding a complete mathematical representation and solution of the problem.

The authors assumed that in the active gas phase region, of extent δ, convection and radiation could be neglected. Thus this region is dominated by diffusion and chemical reaction. An inexplicit solution was obtained for the gas-phase energy equation. That is, instead of completing integration of the non-linear energy equation, a dimensionless analysis approach permitted the equation to be cast in a general functional form. Following differentiation in the direction normal to the surface the heat flux to the fuel surface is represented as:

$$\dot{Q}_s = K(Q_c/C)Y_{ox}F(P,Y_{ox}) \qquad\qquad (4)$$

where K and C are the thermal conductivity and specific heat of the gas-phase respectively, Q_c is the heat released per unit of fuel burned and $F(P,Y_{ox})$ represents the dimensionless integral which is an implicit function of P and Y_{ox}.

11

*Combination of Results from the Gas-Phase Analysis With the
Results From the Solid-Phase Analysis:*

Assuming that the energy conducted into the surface from the gas-phase is equal to the energy conducted away from the surface into the fuel bed, that is, the energy absorbed by surface vaporization is negligible, the right hand side of equation 4 can be combined with the algebraic relationships (equations 1 and 2) derived from the solid-phase energy equation to yield:

Thermally Thin Fuel Bed:

$$V' \simeq \frac{KQ_c Y_{ox} F(P,Y_{ox})}{\rho_s C_s C\tau'(T_b - T_o)} \tag{5}$$

Thermally Thick Fuel Bed:

$$V \simeq \frac{\{KQ_c Y_{ox} F(P,Y_{ox})\}^2}{\rho_s C_s C^2 K_s \delta (T_b - T_o)^2} \tag{6}$$

These simple equations provide a basis for data correlation and design. But theoretically, the approach is unsatisfying in that the actual problem calls for an eigenfunction solution of coupled partial differential equations, but the above equations result from a local heat balance. Further, it involves only the heat flux normal to the direction of flame propagation.

de Ris (11)

de Ris has made a series of assumptions that permits exact mathematical solution of his model. He speculated that the problem could be posed as a gas-phase laminar diffusion flame spreading against an air stream over a solid fuel bed. Both a thin-sheet fuel bed and a semi-infinite fuel bed were considered. (That is, conditions corresponding to thermally thin and thermally thick fuel beds.)

The heat transfer forward to the unburned semi-infinite fuel bed is assumed to take place by conduction through both the gas-phase and fuel bed, as well as by radiation. An exponentially decreasing form for the forward radiative heat transfer is postulated. For simplicity, the thin fuel-bed problem only includes the gas-phase conductive heat transfer. In both cases convective forward heat transfer is zero, since the air stream opposes the flame spread.

The formulated model treats the combustion, which is presumed to take place in the gas-phase, as a diffusion flame that touches the fuel bed at the point where it starts to vaporize. (This approach neglects the existence of a finite ignition region and assumes that the combustion rate is primarily controlled by the mass transfer of reactants to the flame, rather than by the chemical kinetics.) Such a flame can be analyzed employing the Schvab-Zeldovich diffusion flame theory. This approach avoids the effects of highly non-linear reaction kinetics, since the details of the reaction kinetics are ignored by assuming infinite reaction rates in the region of interest.

This diffusion flame approximation is probably valid at distances relatively far from the leading edge of the flame since it is reasonable to expect in this region that the ratio of mass transport time to chemical reaction time, i.e. Damkoler Number [12], is large. However, in the flame attachment region, that is the ignition region which extends over the distance δ, heat loss to the solid and a paucity of fuel vapors must result in a relatively low reaction intensity. Therefore, in this region, the Damkoler Number will be relatively small and hence the diffusion flame assumption is probably invalid.

de Ris's approach resulted in the following flame spread expressions:

Thermally Thin Fuel Bed:

$$V' = \sqrt{2}\ K\ (T_f - T_o)/\rho_s C_s \tau'(T_b - T_o) \tag{7}$$

Thermally Thick Fuel Bed (Neglecting radiation):

$$V = V_a \frac{\rho C K}{\rho_s C_s K_s} \left\{ \frac{T_f - T_b}{T_b - T_o} \right\}^2 \tag{8}$$

where T_f is the flame temperature, V_a is the air velocity with respect to the stationary flame and the other terms are as defined in the previous section.

A comparison of the de Ris flame spread expressions, equations (7) and (8) with those of Lastrina, Magee, and McAlevy equations (5) and (6), reveals that both predict identical dependence on solid phase parameters, e.g. ρ_s, C_s, K_s, τ', and $T_b - T_o$. In addition, recognizing their ignition region, δ, as de Ris's characteristic gas-phase length, i.e.

$$\delta = \frac{2K}{\rho C V_a}$$

and assuming that the group $Q_c/C\ Y_{ox}\ F(P, Y_{ox})$ is proportional to $T_f - T_b$, equations (5) and (6) have been shown to be identical to equations (7), (8) and (2).

Due to the identical representation of the influence of solid phase parameters on flame spread rate predicted by the two approaches, it is concluded that the basic assumption of Lastrina, Magee and McAlevy, that all the processes of interest occur in the small region δ, is well supported. And integration from $-\infty$ to $+\infty$, as was performed by de Ris, is unnecessary.

The differences in assumptions concerning gas phase phenomena of interest are large, and it is perhaps fortuitous that simple substitutions reduce the differences as shown. Until information concerning the structure of the gas phase flame is developed, it appears that it will be impossible to assess the relative validities of the assumptions employed in each analyses.

13

Tarifa, Notario and Torralbo (Reference 13)

Their model of the flame spreading phenomenon considers heating of the fuel ahead of the flame, fuel vaporization and mixing with the oxidizer and flame propagation through this combustible mixture. The flame spreading velocity results from the balance of all these processes.

Their analysis considers that the heat forward from the flame to the unburnt fuel surface is due to radiation only. Starting with an assumed value of the flame spread rate and using an approximate expression for the radiant heat flux from the flame to the fuel, the temperature distribution at the fuel surface is calculated (by an approximate method based on the assumption that heat flux parallel to the fuel surface is small as compared with heat flux perpendicular to the fuel surface). With this temperature distribution and using an assumed vaporization law, the mass conservation equations give the fuel vapor mass fraction at the fuel surface, $Y_{f,s}$. Then, $Y_{f,s}$ was obtained from consideration of the laminar flame speed in the gaseous phase as a function of $Y_{f,s}$. Inasmuch as both approaches for $Y_{f,s}$ are functions of flame velocity, only one flame velocity is found to exist at which the two values of $Y_{f,s}$ match; and this is the flame velocity.

Due to the complexity of the analysis the authors were unable to express the flame velocity analytically in terms of solid and gas-phase parameters. Consequently this approach prohibits designers from extracting the pertinent physical parameters governing flame propagation, and researchers from checking the theoretical predictions against experimental results.

EXPERIMENTS — RESULTS — CONCLUSIONS

This section is organized in segments in which, successively, some experiments by the authors as well as other investigators, the results from these experiments and their comparison with the predictions of the three major flame spread theories are presented.

Flame Spread Over Thermally Thick Fuel Beds

All the data obtained to date in the authors' laboratory, of flame spread rate over thermally thick fuel beds can be correlated by a universal power-law relationship between the flame spreading velocity (V) and two gas-phase parameters, pressure (P) and oxygen mole fraction (Y_{ox}). The apparatus and experimental procedure employed are described in Reference 1.

Specifically, the influence of P on V for two thermoplastics, polystyrene and polymethylmethacrylate, for various values of Y_{ox} in O_2/N_2 and O_2/H_e environments is shown in Figures 1 and 2 respectively. The measured flame spreading velocity in all cases could be correlated, over a pressure range of 400 psia, with the test-gas environmental parameters Y_{ox} and P (see Figures 3 and 4) in the form

$$V \propto (PY_{ox}^m)^\Phi$$

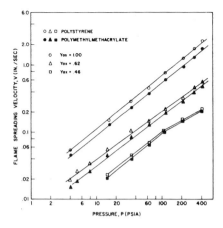

Figure 1. *V VS P for two thermoplastics in* O_2/N_2 *environments.*

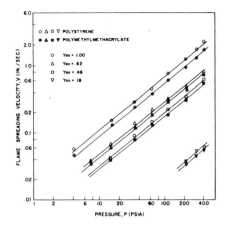

Figure 2. *V VS P for two thermoplastics in* O_2/He *environments.*

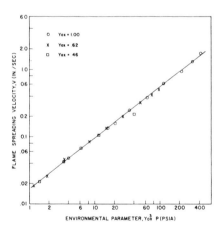

Figure 3. *V VS* $Y_{ox}^3 P$ *for polymethylmethacrylate in* O_2/N_2 *environments.*

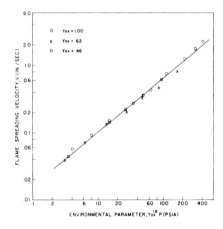

Figure 4. *V VS* $Y_{ox}^{1.9} P$ *for polystyrene in* O_2/He *environments.*

as predicted by McAlevy and Magee [1]. Nitrate ester propellant data could also be correlated by this equation over the same pressure range. Experimentally determined values of Φ and m are shown in Table 7.

Due to the fact that the systems tested had widely varying chemical properties, a general conclusion can be drawn from the successful correlation of all these data by the same equation: V is controlled by a common, gas-phase, physical process — probably either heat or mass transfer.

15

Inspection of Table 7 reveals that m is a function of diluent gas and type of specimen, either thermoplastic or solid propellant, while Φ, although dependent upon the type of specimen, is relatively insensitive to the diluent gas. The simplified analysis of McAlevy and Magee [1] resulted in the correct prediction of the functional dependence of V upon P and Y_{ox} and allowed qualitative predictions to be made regarding Φ and m. However, it resulted in poor quantitative predictions.

Flame Spreading Characteristics of Thin and Thick Cellulosic Specimens

The flame-spreading velocity over the surface of cellulosic specimens was measured in quiescent environments of various pressures and compositions by Royal [19]. The apparatus and experimental procedure employed are described in Reference 1. Test specimens were fabricated from 3 x 5 inch, white unruled index cards, 0.0088 in. thick. Specimens of varying thickness were made by a lamination technique. Individual cards were soaked in water, superposed on each other, and pressed together at a nominal pressure of 15,000 psi. The specimens were allowed to room-dry overnight and then dried for at least one hour in an oven at 220 F. Single cards were also dried to remove any moisture they might have absorbed. The specimens were mounted vertically in an asbestos holder which inhibited the edge-effect noted previously [1, 3]. The specimens were then ignited at the top and the flame spread evenly down both sides.

Figure 5 shows the effect of varying thickness on the flame spreading velocity in air at one atmosphere. Over a substantial range of the thicknesses tested (0.0088 in. to 0.077 in.), the flame spreading velocity varies inversely with the specimen thickness as predicted by Lastrina *et al* and de Ris [2, 11]. For specimens thicker than 0.060 in., or so, there is an indication that V is less sensitive to thickness. Unfortunately, it was not possible to obtain data for thicker samples at these environmental conditions, as the flame appeared to become unstable and quenched after ignition.

Further tests were performed with single card specimens and the results plotted in Figure 6. Equation 3 was employed to calculate the shaded area ($\bar{\tau} \simeq 1$) between

Table 7. Experimental Values of Φ and m.

Specimen	Environmental composition					
	O_2/N_2		O_2/He		O_2/Ar	
	Φ	m	Φ	m	Φ	m
Propellant A	0.62	2 ·	—	—	—	—
Propellant B	0.65	2	—	—	—	—
Polystyrene	0.76	3	0.80	1.9	0.83	2.6
Polymethylmethacrylate	0.82	3	0.78	1.9	0.78	2.6

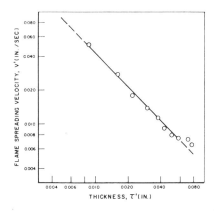

Figure 5. *V'VS τ' for thin cellulosic specimens in air at one atmosphere.*

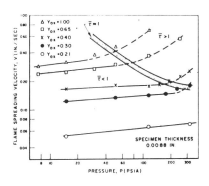

Figure 6. *V'VS P for thin cellulosic specimens in O_2/N_2 environments.*

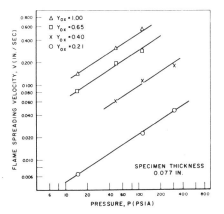

Figure 7. *V VS P for thick cellulosic specimens in O_2/N_2 environments.*

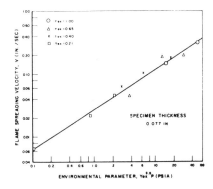

Figure 8. *V VS $Y_{ox}^{3.3} P$ for thick cellulosic specimens in O_2/N_2 environments.*

the regime of thermally thin fuel bed flame spreading characteristics ($\bar{\tau} < 1$) and thermally thick fuel bed characteristics ($\bar{\tau} > 1$). The data support the validity of this criterion. In the region of thermally thin fuel bed characteristics, $V'(P, Y_{ox})$ is well represented by means of a power-law. The pressure exponent is small (ranging between 0.05 and 0.1) — but not zero as predicted by de Ris [11] — while the dependence on Y_{ox} is much stronger ($V' \sim Y_{ox}^{0.9}$).

In the region of thermally thick fuel bed characteristics, experiments with laminated specimens ($\tau = 0.077$ in.) indicated that $V(P, Y_{ox}) \sim Y_{ox}^{2.1} P^{.63}$. These data are represented in Figures 7 and 8. The data of Figure 6 and Figure 7 can be used to obtain information concerning $F(P, Y_{ox})$. This function appears in both equation 5

17

and equation 6. Since equation 5 predicts $V' \propto Y_{ox} F(P,Y_{ox})$, and the data in Figure 6 can be correlated by $V' \propto Y_{ox}^{0.9} P^{0.05}$, $F(P,Y_{ox})$ is a very weak function of P and Y_{ox}. From previous measurements on thick fuel beds it was found that $\delta \sim P^{-0.5}$. Thus equation 6 can be written as $V \propto Y_{ox}^2 P^{0.5} F(P,Y_{ox})^2$. Comparison with the empirical power-law $V \propto Y_{ox}^{2.1} P^{.63}$ indicates again that $F(P,Y_{ox})$ is a very weak function of P and Y_{ox}. For other materials and environmental conditions this dependence might change somewhat. Unfortunately, data for *both* thin and thick specimens of materials other than cellulose are nonexistent. However, data obtained previously for thick polymethylmethacrylate (PMM) specimens in O_2/N_2 environments, indicated $V \propto Y_{ox}^{2.4} P^{.82}$. This suggests that $F(P,Y_{ox}) \propto Y_{ox}^{.23} P^{.16}$ for PMM, a dependence slightly different than that for cellulose. It is believed, in the case of cellulose, that a combination of data scatter and curve fitting errors accounts for the discrepancy of the Y_{ox} dependence of $F(P,Y_{ox})$. (In the case of thin fuel bed the exponent $\simeq -0.1$, while for thick beds, the exponent $\simeq 0.05$).

The ability to successfully correlate the observed flame spreading characteristics of both the thin and thick cellulosic fuel beds, tends to verify the validity of flame spreading equations 5 and 6. However, de Ris has shown that his theoretical results correlate the data equally as well [2]. The reader is referred to the Theory Section for further discussion of this commonality and its probable fortuitous nature.

Flame Spreading Over Various Materials — Thin and Thick Fuel Specimens

The influence of oxygen concentration on flame propagation over a variety of fuel materials in quiescent environments was obtained experimentally by Huggett *et al* [6]. These authors attempted to correlate the flame spreading velocity with the logarithm of the specific heat of the gas mixture divided by the oxygen mole fraction, i.e. $V \propto \log (C/Y_{ox})$. Figure 9 which shows typical data obtained by Huggett *et al* demonstrates that the flame spreading data can also be correlated equally well by $V \propto (C/Y_{ox})^{-b}$.

According to equations 5 and 6, and the results reported for cellulose which implied that $F(P,Y_{ox})$ is a weak function of P and Y_{ox}, V should be proportional to $(C/Y_{ox})^{-b}$ where $b \simeq 1.0$ for thin fuel specimens and $b \simeq 2.0$ for thick fuel specimens. Table 8 lists the type and thickness of the fuel specimen, the empirical exponent b, and the theoretically predicted exponent b. These results, which were not interpreted in this fashion by Huggett *et al*, are generally consistent with the dependencies of thin and thick fuel beds on oxygen concentration and specific heat of the gas mixture as predicted by Lastrina, Magee and McAlevy [2].

Effect of Preheating the Unburnt Fuel Bed by a Radiation Source

The influence on flame propagation of preheating the unburnt fuel bed was investigated by G. K. Kwentus in both quiescent and convective flow environments [20]. The fuel bed (12 in. wide by 4 ft. long) consisted of a layer of tamped shredded newsprint (approximately 0.02 in. thick) placed on top of an insulating fiberglass base. The flame velocity was obtained for various total radiant heat fluxes

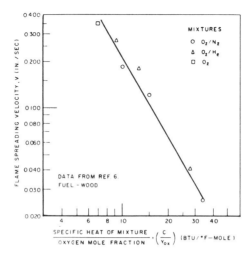

Figure 9. *V VS (C/Y$_{ox}$) for various O$_2$/inert mixtures.*

Table 8. *Comparison of Experimental and Predicted Exponent of Y$_{ox}$ for Thin and Thick Fuel Beds.*

Fuel Specimen		Empirical Exponent*	Predicted Exponent**
Material	Thickness (in.)	b	b
paper	0.008	0.96	1.0
painted surface	0.016	0.91	1.0
foam cushion	0.250	2.06	2.0
wood	0.066	1.74	transition thickness
cellulose acetate	0.250	1.27	2.0

 * Data from Reference 6.
 ** b≃1 for thin fuel specimens; b≃2 for thick fuel specimens.

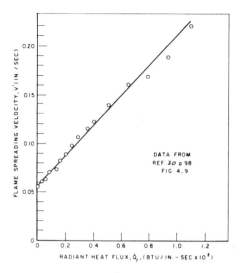

Figure 10. V' VS $\dot{Q}_r$ for shredded newsprint thin fuel bed.

striking the unburnt fuel bed and for various environmental conditions. Typical data of flame velocity (V) versus total radiant heat flux ($\dot{Q}_r$) are shown in Figure 10. Values of the slopes of V versus $\dot{Q}_r$ varied from 11 in^2/Btu to 20 in^2/Btu depending on environmental conditions.

For this experiment, the total heat flux to the unburnt fuel surface is made up of a normal heat flux from the flame ($\dot{Q}_s$) plus the heat flux from the controlled radiation source ($\dot{Q}_r$). Extending the thin fuel bed analysis* of Lastrina, Magee and McAlevy (Equation 1) for the case of two independent heat fluxes to the surface, it is apparent that:

$$\rho_s C_s V' \tau' (T_b - T_o) = \dot{Q}_r + \dot{Q}_s$$

or

$$\frac{dV'}{d\dot{Q}_r} = \frac{1}{\rho_s C_s \tau' (T_b - T_o)}$$

The above analysis predicts the flame velocity should increase linearly with the radiant heat flux; and the slope of this line should equal $1/\rho_s C_s \tau' (T_b - T_o)$. Using appropriate values for $\rho_s \tau'$, C_s, and $(T_b - T_o)$, the value of the slope is approximately 11 in^2/Btu [16]. Thus the subject data support the analytical predictions of the Stevens group.

---

*The validity of assuming a thin fuel bed cannot be verified since the magnitude of δ, required to determine the critical thickness separating thin from thick fuel beds, is not reported by Kwentus. The thickness of the fuel (0.02 in.) is less than the critical thickness of cellulosic specimens 0.03 in.

Influence of Initial Temperature on Flame Spreading Velocity

The influence of the initial temperature of the solid on flame spreading velocity in a quiescent environment was investigated for both PMM and cellulosic specimens by Bhat [21]. However, a different experimental procedure was employed for each material.

In the case of PMM, 1/8" thick samples of the solid (3/8" x 3") were mounted horizontally in a test chamber [1]. The chamber was charged with oxygen at atmospheric pressure and the temperature of the top surface, i.e. the flame spreading surface, was raised to the desired value (up to 140 C) by conductive heating from a strip-heater fastened to the specimen bottom surface. Thermal gradients normal to the surface were minimized by employing relatively long heating times, e.g. 15 min. The sample was then ignited by an electrically heated wire.

The cellulosic specimens were mounted vertically in an asbestos holder, placed in an isothermal oven (18 x 18 x 15 in.) and heated to the desired temperature (up to 210 C). Once the specimen achieved thermal equilibrium with the surroundings, it was ignited at the top and the flame spread down both sides. Hence, both specimen and environment were at elevated temperature. Both thin (0.0088 in.) and thick (0.077 in.) cellulosic specimens, identical to those referred to earlier were tested.

The data obtained from these experiments were correlated using the relationship,

$$V \propto (T_b - T_o)^{-n}$$

as suggested by equations 5, 6, 7 and 8, to obtain empirical values of n. This required knowledge of T_b for both materials. Values of T_b have been obtained for PMM (400 C − Reference 1) and cellulose (370 C for thermally thin specimens and 420 C for thermally thick specimens, Reference 21).

Employing a value of T_b = 400 C, the PMM data obtained were plotted on a graph of 1n V vs 1n $(T_b - T_o)$ (Figure 12). A "least squares" fit of the data yielded a value of n = 1.95, which is in close agreement with the theoretical prediction of n = 2 for thermally thick fuel beds. Hence, these results seem to verify the theoretical predictions regarding the influence of initial fuel bed temperature on the flame spreading velocity over thermally thick fuel beds.

Bhat also compared his data with the PMM data reported by Tarifa, *et al* [13], as shown in Figure 11. They observed a sudden increase in the flame spreading velocity, of the order of two magnitudes, above an initial temperature of about 100 C. This was not observed by Bhat. The difference between the flame spreading rates reported by Tarifa *et al* and those measured by Bhat are probably a result of the difference in the geometries and preparation of the specimens tested. Tarifa *et al* employed PMM rods, heated from the center by an electrical wire, and measured the downward vertical flame spread rate. However, they also employed horizontal strips at temperatures above 90–100 C. And the edges of these strips were not reported to be inhibited. Therefore, it is assumed that the high flame spread rates measured above 100 C are a result of the rapid edge-burning phenomenon reported by McAlevy and Magee [1, 3], and are not the actual flame spreading velocities at those conditions.

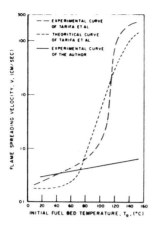

Figure 11. *Log V VS T_o for thick poly-methylmethacrylate specimens in oxygen at one atmosphere.*

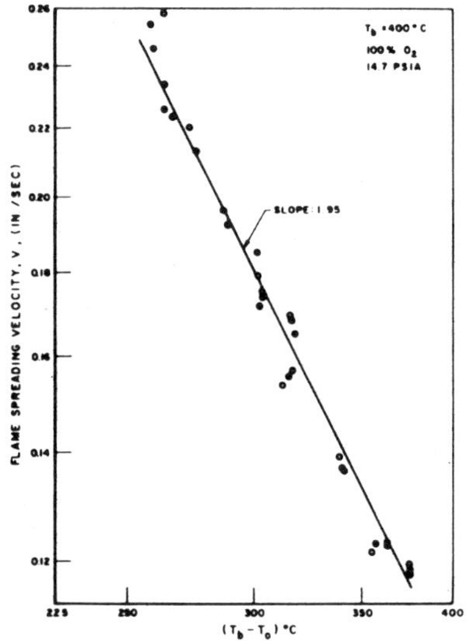

Figure 12. *Log V VS log $(T_b - T_o)$ for thick polymethylmethacrylate specimens.*

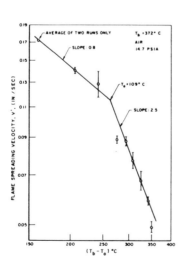
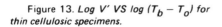

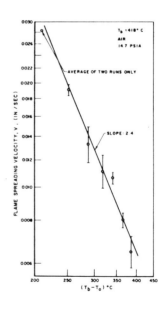

Figure 13. *Log V' VS log $(T_b - T_o)$ for thin cellulosic specimens.*

Figure 14. *Log V VS log $(T_b - T_o)$ for thick cellulosic specimens.*

Figures 13 and 14 are plots of 1n V vs 1n (T_b-T_o) for thermally thin and thermally thick cellulosic specimens respectively. The thermally thin cellulosic result, n = 2.5, contradicts the theoretical predictions (Equations 5, 7) n = 1.0. Also the slope of the curve changes above T_o = 110 C. For the thermally thick cellulosic specimens, the data yields n = 2.4 which compares favorably with the theoretically predicted exponent 2.0. However, this may be fortuitous since there seems to be little difference in the dependency of flame spreading velocity on initial temperature for thin and thick fuel beds below T_o = 110 C.

Deviation from prediction for cellulosic specimens might be a result of their decomposition process. For while PMM may be thought to undergo a simple surface decomposition-vaporization process upon application of surface heating, there is evidence that cellulosic materials undergo decomposition in depth [23]. Thus, the PMM data, and to a lesser extent the thick cellulosic data, support the analysis of Lastrina *et al* and de Ris. But more information concerning the transient thermal decomposition characteristics of cellulosic materials is required before the thin specimen data can be rationalized.

Flame Spreading in Convective Flow Environments Opposed To The Flame Spread

Experimentally, the influence on flame propagation of forced convective motion opposed to the flame spread of environments composed of various inert gases and oxygen mole fractions was investigated by Lastrina [16].

Experiments were performed in a "blow-down" wind tunnel, driven by high-pressure, bottled test gas. The test section geometry was 1" x 1" x 12". The test gas (O_2/inert mixtures) was admitted through 5 manifold-holes located in the head-end, and swept over 1/8" thick, flush-mounted, test specimens (3/8" wide x 4" long), located along the centerline with the leading edge 4" from the head-end of the test section. An inorganic cement was used along the specimen sides to insure that the propagating flame remained planar. The back-end of the tunnel was open to the atmosphere. No attempt was made to measure the velocity profile over the specimen. Instead, the mean flow velocity was calculated from measured mass flow rates by means of the continuity equation.

Specimens were ignited by an electrically heated wire (certain conditions required the use of an easily-ignited ignition charge) at the back end. Flame spreading velocity data was taken over the middle two inches. Polymethylmethacrylate (PMM) and polyurethane were subjected to test. Typical data are shown in Figure 15.

All data exhibited increasing flame propagation velocity with increasing flow velocity until a "critical" flow velocity was reached. All of the data obtained below the critical flow velocity could be correlated by the empirical power-law relationship:

$$V \propto U^{.34} Y_{ox}^d$$

where U is the test gas flow velocity. (This finding contrasts with the de Ris prediction of $V \propto U$.) Values of "d" for both quiescent and forced convective environments are listed in Table 9. The empirical dependence of V on Y_{ox} appears to be identical in both the quiescent and forced convective environments.

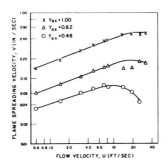

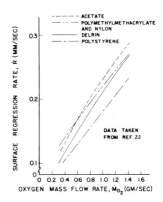

Figure 15. *V VS U for thick PMM fuel specimens in O_2/N_2 environments.*

Figure 16. *Linear pyrolysis characteristics.*

Table 9. *Experimental Values of d.*

	PMM		POLYURETHANE	
	Quiescent d*	Convective d	Quiescent d	Convective d
O_2/N_2	2.46	1.94	1.95	2.07
O_2/Ar	2.03	2.04	–	2.17
O_2/He	1.48	1.36	–	1.52

* Reference 1.

To investigate further the influence of forced convective motion on flame propagation below the critical flow velocity, Lastrina made a limited number of surface temperature profile measurements (at least three tests were performed at each of four values of U) using the techniques reported in Reference 1, with PMM in 46% O_2, 54% Ar. Experimentally, δ was found to vary with U in a way that can be correlated by the empirical power-law $\delta \propto U^{-1/3}$. For this result to be consistent with the observed flame spreading dependence on flow velocity and Equation 2; $\dot{Q}_s$ is required to be essentially independent of the flow velocity. Results from the numerical work demonstrated this fact [16].

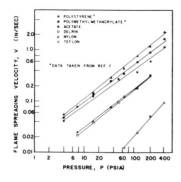

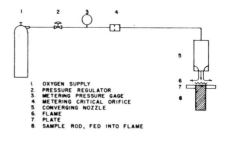

Figure 17. *V VS P for various test materials in 100% O₂ environment.*

Figure 18. *Schematic of apparatus for linear pyrolysis measurement employed in Reference 22.*

Effect of Quasi-Steady Linear Pyrolysis Characteristics on Flame Spreading Velocity

The transient surface vaporization process is a pivotally important boundary condition in any flame spread model. However, transient surface pyrolysis characteristics are unknown. Baham, therefore, attempted to correlate the flame spread rate with available quasi-steady pyrolysis characteristics [4].

Figures 16 and 17 were employed by Baham to determine whether or not a correlation of quasi-steady state linear pyrolysis characteristics with flame spreading velocity exists. Figure 16 shows linear pyrolysis data for several materials taken from Reference 22, and the schematic arrangement of the apparatus employed to obtain this pyrolysis data is shown in Figure 18. Figure 17 shows the corresponding flame spread velocity data of Baham. From an examination of Figures 16 and 17 it is clear that there is no correlation of flame spreading velocity with quasi-steady linear pyrolysis characteristics for the materials tested.

SUMMARY

With the exception of the influence of initial temperature on flame spread rate, most data from well-defined laboratory experiments can be correlated on the basis of equations derived by the Stevens group. However, as indicated in the Theory section, their equations can be shown to be similar to the de Ris equations after making a series of additional assumptions. Thus, the more valid approach cannot be discerned on this basis; the basic assumptions of each model must be tested. Since the flame zone structure itself has never been studied, there is no experimental evidence against which the assumed models can be compared. And an impasse exists at this time. It can be broken only by the weight of new evidence concerning the flame zone structure, not by additional theorizing.

REFERENCES

1. R. F. McAlevy, III and R. S. Magee, "The Mechanism of Flame Spreading over the Surface of Igniting, Condensed Phase Materials" *Twelfth Symposium (International) on Combustion,* The Combustion Institute, 1969, p. 215.

2. F. A. Lastrina, R. S. Magee, and R. F. McAlevy, III, "Flame Spread Over Fuel Beds: Solid Phase Energy Considerations," *Thirteenth Symposium (International) on Combustion,* The Combustion Institute, 1971, p. 935.

3. R. F. McAlevy, III, R. S. Magee, P. M. Baham and F. A. Lastrina, "Some Recent Experimental Observations on Flame Spreading Over Solid Fuel Surfaces", Presented at the 1969 Fall Meeting, Western States Section, The Combustion Institute, 27-28 Oct., LaJolla, California.

4. P. M. Baham, "Diagnostic Tests of Some Models of Flame Spreading Over Condensed Phase Materials", Master Thesis, Stevens Institute of Technology, 1969.

5. C. Huggett, G. von Elbe, W. Haggerty, and J. Grossman, "The Effects of 100% Oxygen at Reduced Pressure on the Ignitibility and Combustibility of Materials," Brooks Air Force Base, Report SAM-TR-65-78, December 1965. Prepared by Atlantic Research Corporation.

6. C. Huggett, G. von Elbe, and W. Haggerty, "The Combustibility of Materials in Oxygen-Helium and Oxygen-Nitrogen Atmospheres," Brooks Air Force Base, Report SAM-TR-66-85, December 1966. Prepared by Atlantic Research Corporation.

7. J. E. Johnson, and F. J. Woods, "Flammability in Unusual Atmospheres. Part 1 — Preliminary Studies of Materials in Hyperbaric Atmospheres Containing Oxygen, Nitrogen, and/or Helium," Naval Research Laboratory, Washington, D. C., Report 6470, 1966.

8. G. A. Cook, R. E. Meierer, and B. M. Shields, "Screening of Flame-Resistant Materials and Comparison of Helium with Nitrogen for Use in Diving Atmospheres," Linde Division, Union Carbide Corporation, Tonawanda, New York, March 1967. Prepared for ONR under Contract No. N00014-66-C0149.

9. R. C. Rothermel, and H. E. Anderson, "Fire Spread Characteristics Determined in the Laboratory," U. S. Forest Service, Research Paper INT-30, 1966. Inter-mountain Forest & Range Experiment Station, Ogden, Utah.

10. R. Friedman, "A Survey of Knowledge About Idealized Fire Spread Over Surfaces," *Fire Research Abstracts and Reviews,* 10, 1968, p. 1.

11. J. N. de Ris, "The Spread of a Laminar Diffusion Flame" *Twelfth Symposium (International) on Combustion,* The Combustion Institute, 1969, p. 241.

12. C. H. Waldmen, S. I. Cheng, W. A. Sirignano, and M. Summerfield, "Theoretical Studies of Diffusion Flame Structures," AMS Report No. 860, AFOSR CONTRACT AF 49 (638) 1267, Jan. 1969.

13. C. S. Tarifa, P. P. Notario, A. M. Torralbo, "On the Process of Flame Spreading Over the Surface of Plastic Fuels in an Oxidizing Atmosphere" *Twelfth Symposium (International) on Combustion,* The Combustion Institute, 1969, p. 229.

14. W. J. Parker, "Flame Spread Model For Cellulosic Materials," Presented at the March 1969 Meeting, Central States Section, The Combustion Institute, University of Minnesota.

15. J. A. Wrubel, "Flame Spreading Over the Surface of Double Base Propellants at High Pressure" Masters Thesis, Stevens Institute of Technology, Hoboken, New Jersey, June 1966.

16. F. A. Lastrina, "Flame Spread Over Solid Fuel Beds, Solid and Gas Phase Energy Considerations," Ph.D. Thesis, Stevens Institute of Technology, June 1970.

17. W. J. Most, and M. Summerfield, "Starting Thrust Transients of Solid Rocket Engines" Aeospace and Mechanical Sciences Report No. 873, Princeton University, Princeton, N. J., July 1969.

18. R. S. Magee, "The Mechanism of Flame Spreading Over The Surface of Igniting Condensed Phase Materials" D.Sc. Thesis, Stevens Institute of Technology, 1968.

19. J. H. Royal, "The Influence of Fuel Bed Thickness On Flame Spreading Rate," Honors Report, Stevens Institute of Technology, 1970.

20. G. K. Kwentus, "Fuel Preheating in Free-Burning Fires," Ph.D. Thesis, Massachusetts Institute of Technology, 1967.

21. P. R. Bhat, "Influence of Initial Fuel Bed Temperature on Flame Spreading Velocity" Masters Thesis, Stevens Institute of Technology, 1970.

22. J. V. Havel, "The Linear Pyrolysis of Several Thermoplastics During Combustion" Masters Thesis, Stevens Institute of Technology, June 1969.

23. K. A. Murty, and P. L. Blackshear, Jr., "An X-Ray Photographic Study of the Reaction Kinetics of α-Cellulose Decomposition," Western States Section, The Combustion Institute, April 1966.

Presented at the 1971 Polymer Conference Series, Flammability Characteristics of Polymeric Materials Conference at the University of Utah.

R. S. Magee

Richard S. Magee is an Associate Professor of Mechanical Engineering at Stevens Institute of Technology in Hoboken, New Jersey. He received his B.E., M.S., and Sc.D. degrees from Stevens Institute of Technology in 1963, 1964, and 1968, respectively. He has been involved in combustion research since 1963, much of it related to flame spreading over the surface of combustible materials.

R. F. McAlevy III

Robert F. McAlevy III is a Professor of Mechanical Engineering and Director of the Combustion Laboratory at Stevens Institute of Technology at Hoboken, New Jersey. He received his M.E. degree from Stevens Institute of Technology in 1954 and his Ph.D. degree in Aeronautical Engineering from Princeton University in 1960. His research work has covered various aspects of combustion.

Flame Spread Rates of Solid Combustibles in Compressed and Oxygen-Enriched Atmospheres

Atsushi Nakakuki

Fire Research Institute
Mitaka, Tokyo, Japan

(Received September 3, 1971)

ABSTRACT

The flame-spread rates of various solid combustibles in a vessel of volume 9.2 m^3 in compressed and oxygen-enriched atmospheres were measured. The flame-spread rates were obtained under conditions where buoyancy effects were not so large. They depended upon the convective current of the ambient gas. The flame-spread rates of samples supported at their ends only were found to be proportional to the product of both powers of oxygen concentration and total pressure, and to depend far more upon oxygen concentration than upon total pressure when compared at the same oxygen partial pressure.

INTRODUCTION

The information concerning flame-spread rates under hyperbaric conditions has been rather limited until recently [1, 2, 3, 4]. The flame-spread rate of a solid combustible can vary largely with the angle at which the material is set because of buoyancy effects. The buoyancy effects increase with the angle when the direction of burning is upward and are especially noticeable when the sample is flamed up. The angle of 45° with upward burning is frequently used to determine the flame-spread rate of highly fire resistant materials, but is not necessarily appropriate for common materials. Therefore, in this investigation, the angle was selected according to the type of material, and flame-spread rates were determined for several combustible materials in air and various oxygen-nitrogen atmospheres at pressures from 1 to 3 atmospheres.

EXPERIMENTAL

The pressure vessel used for these experiments was 2 m in I.D. by about 3 m long. The vessel was equipped with six glass observation windows. The oxygen concentration in the vessel was made uniform as quickly as possible by discharging oxygen from 14 holes at the inner wall of the vessel. The air was sent to the vessel through a dehumidifier by an oil-free compressor.

Flame-spread rates of single combustible samples were measured and the appearance of the flame spread was observed. The sample was ignited at one end by an n-hexane flame or an electrically heated coil of nichrome wire. N-hexane was ignited by an electric spark. The time of flame spread from one end of the sample to the other one was measured directly with a stop watch or by photographing with a 16 mm motion picture camera. The volume of burning products of the sample was so small compared with that of the vessel that gas composition in the vessel varied little during combustion.

Combustible samples used were cypress (Japanese), rayon white cloth (standardized for dyeing test by the Japanese Industrial Standard), PVC coated electric wire — vinyl cord (2×0.75 mm^2), filter paper (No. 2), and pig's flesh and skin. In the case of rayon cloth and filter paper, the rectangular sample 40 cm long was fixed at its lengthwise ends to the rectangular steel frame. Samples of the pig's flesh and skin were also rectangular and c.a. 20 cm long, and fixed to the same frame. The wood sample of square section was fixed at one end to support and ignited at the other end. The sample of vinyl cord was fixed at both ends to the supports.

In these experiments, the angles at which the samples were mounted were varied with the type of material properly, and kept small enough to minimize the flame size and the buoyancy effects.

RESULTS AND DISCUSSIONS

Table 1 gives data for the filter paper and Table 2 those for the cypress burnt at various dimensions and angles in various atmospheres. Each value in these tables is the average of 3 experiments. As expected, with the increase of the angle with

Table 1. Flame-Spread Rate of Filter Paper (No. 2 — Effect of Sample Dimension (1)

Mode of Burning	Ambient pressure (atm abs.)	Oxygen Concentration (%)	Flame-Spread Rate (em/sec)		
			Sample dimension Width × Length (mm)		
			20 × 400	40 × 400	100 × 400
45° Angle	1	21	0.13	0.12	0.14
		40	0.54	0.55	0.52
Downward	3	21	0.19	0.20	0.18
Horizontal	1	21	0.17	0.19	0.23
		40	0.62	0.70	1.5
	3	21	0.35	0.55	0.95
45° Angle	1	21	1.5	1.9	2.7
		40	3.2	4.4	6.7
Upward	3	21	3.0	4.1	4.8

upward or downward burning, the flame-spread rate increases or decreases respectively. It increases with air pressure and oxygen concentration, and more when the oxygen concentration is increased than when the air pressure is increased. Under the same atmosphere, the flame-spread rate for the filter paper does not vary with the sample width at the angle of 45° with downward burning, but increases at the horizontal and 45° with upward burning due to the increase of buoyancy effect and flame size with the sample width. Particularly at the angle of 45° with upward burning, the correct spread rate could not be measured for material of high flame-spread rate, e.g. rayon cloth, because the flame became large and contacted the unburned material above it. For the filter paper and rayon cloth, the flame spreads faster at both edges of the sample than at the center, because the convection of the ambient fresh gas is greater at the side edges. When the sample was also fixed at both side edges to the frame, the flame spread became far slower on account of the interruption of the convection at side edges. For wood samples, flame-spread rates increase with the decrease of the sectional area as seen from Table 3. The flame becomes large at the underneath side of the sample especially in oxygen-enriched atmospheres as shown in Figure 1, because fresh gas contacts the underneath side and the combustion products flow upward, interrupting the burning process. The same phenomenon was also observed with the vinyl cord.

Wood samples immersed in water for a long time could propagate the flame in the high oxygen atmosphere. Its rate of flame spread is very small compared with the dry sample and decreases with increase of immersion time. The rate of decrease of

Table 2. Flame-Spread Rate of Cypress — Effect of Sample Dimension (2)
Sign ✕ *Shows that Flame Self-extinguished Before Sample was entirely Burned Up*

Mode of Burning	Ambient pressure (atm abs.)	Oxygen Concentration (%)	Flame-Spread Rate (cm/sec) Sample dimension Section ✕ Length (mm)	
			4 ✕ 4 ✕ 200	8 ✕ 8 ✕ 300
Horizontal	1	21	✕	✕
		30	0.20	0.15
		40	0.32	0.32
		50	0.74	0.47
		60	0.82	0.59
	3	21	0.16	✕
45° Angle Upward	1	21	0.16	✕
		30	0.38	0.37
		40	0.74	0.50
		50	0.83	0.58
		60		0.97
	3	21	0.36	0.18

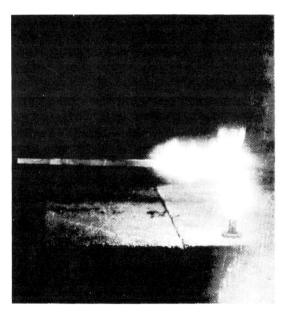

Figure 1. *Flame spread in cypress with horizontal burning at oxygen concentration of 60% under atmospheric pressure. Flame propagates faster in the underneath side.*

the flame-spread rate decreases with the immersion time as seen from Tables 2 and 3. Material which burns so rapidly that there is no time to dry the unburned nearby part does not propagate the flame. For example, the rayon cloth and filter paper immersed in water ignited only at the portion contacted by the flame, and did not propagate the flame.

Table 3. *Flame-Spread Rate of Cypress Immersed in Water at Atmospheric Pressure. Mode of Burning: Horizontal*

Oxygen Concentration (%)	Dimension Section X Length (mm)	Immersed Time (hrs)	Flame-Spread Rate (cm/sec)
50	4 X 4 X 200	24	0.24
60	4 X 4 X 200	24	0.56
30	8 X 8 X 300	1	0.08
40	8 X 8 X 300	1	0.09
50	8 X 8 X 300	1	0.16
30	8 X 8 X 300	24	0.04
40	8 X 8 X 300	24	0.09
50	8 X 8 X 300	24	0.10
60	8 X 8 X 300	24	0.11

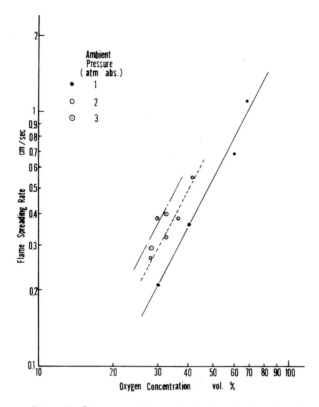

Figure 2. *Flame spread rate of vinyl cord plotted against oxygen concentrates taking total pressure as the parameter.*

Figure 2 is the flame-spread rate of the vinyl cord plotted against the partial pressure of oxygen. Points at each total pressure are approximately linear on the logarithmic plot. These lines are mutually parallel. For results such as in Figure 2, the flame spread rate v (cm/sec) is expressed as follows:

$$v = A \, c^m \, p^n \qquad (1)$$

where c is the volume ratio of oxygen, p is the ambient pressure (atm abs.), and A is the flame-spread rate of p = 1 atm abs, and c = 1 or the oxygen concentration of 100%. McAlevy, et al [5, 6] measured the flame-spreading rate over the surface of various thermoplastics and solid-rocket propellants mounted smooth surface upwards, on backing plates. They found the same relation as Equation (1) and determined the values of m and n. The values of A m and n obtained in this experiment are shown in Table 4. The pressure range which was used in determination of n is shown in the last column of the table. For the rayon cloth and filter paper, flame-spread rates did not vary with the total pressure above 2 atm abs. The values of m and n vary little with the angle of burning in the range of small buoyancy effect as seen in the measurement examples of vinyl cord and filter paper. However, they vary with the type of material. The ratios of m to n are in the range of 2 to 4 as shown at the sixth column of Table 4. Therefore, it is seen that flame-spread rates depend far more upon oxygen concentration than upon total pressure. This fact is different from the customary idea concerning the flame-spread rate of solid combustibles supported at their ends only that it is principally dependent upon the oxygen partial pressure.

The fat which is scattered in the pig-flesh burned with a blue flame, but the flesh itself did not burn. In the case of the skin, the flame spreads very fast hair to hair and then the skin propagates the flame slowly. The flame-spread rates of these materials are shown in Table 5. With the position of the skin, the flame-spread rate varies greatly even at the same oxygen concentration perhaps due to the difference of fat or water content [7].

Table 4. Values of A, m and n

Material	Mode of Burning	A (cm/sec)	m	n	m/n	Pressure Range Applicable (atm abs.)
Cypress	Horizontal	2.63	2.45	0.71	3.45	1 ~ 3
Rayon Cloth	45°, Downward	19.2	2.80	0.73	3.84	1 ~ 2
Vinyl Cord	Horizontal	1.74	1.99	0.52	3.83	1 ~ 3
	45°, Upward	2.02	1.88	0.53	3.55	
Filter Paper	45°, Downward	2.19	1.66	0.75	2.21	1 ~ 2
	Horizontal	2.54	1.59	0.60	2.65	

Table 5. Flame-Spread Rate of Pig-Flesh and-Skin under Atmospheric Pressure at the Angle of 45° with Upward Burning

Material	Oxygen Concentration (%)	Dimension Width (mm)	Length (mm)	Weight (g)	Flame-Spread Rate (cm/sec)
Flesh	70	20	150	50	not ignited
Skin	50	50	300	80	0.044
	50	20	200	40	0.44
	70	20	200	31	1.33
	70	23	200	36	0.80

CONCLUSION

Flame-spread rates of various solid combustibles supported at their ends were measured at various angles. The flame-spread rate increased with pressure and oxygen concentration, and is expressed by the function of the product of both powers of oxygen concentration and total pressure as confirmed already in the flame-spread measurement of various thermoplastics fixed on the backing plate. In the above relation, the ratio of the power of oxygen concentration to that of total pressure was in the range of 2 to 4. Therefore, it can be said that, at the same oxygen partial pressure, the flame-spread rate depends unexpectedly far more upon oxygen concentration than upon total pressure.

REFERENCES

1. J. M. Kuchta, A. L. Furno, and G. H. Martindill, Fire Technology, *5*, 203 (1969).
2. J. E. Johnson, and F. J. Wood, NRL Report 6470 (Oct. 1966), NRL Report 6606 (Sept. 1967).
3. G. A. Cook, R. E. Meierer, and B. M. Shields, Textile Research J., *37*, 591 (1967).
4. D. W. Denison, and J. Ernstrong, FPRC/1249, RAF Institute of Aviation Medicine, Farnsborough, Hants., England (1966).
5. R. F. McAlevy, and R. S. Magee, Twelfth Symp. (International) on Combustion, Combustion Institute, p. 215 (1960).
6. R. F. McAlevy, and R. S. Magee, J. Spacecraft Rockets, *4*, 1390 (1967).
7. R. L. Durfee, SAM-TR-68-130, Aerospace Medical Division, Texas (1968).

Atsushi Nakakuki

Atsushi Nakakuki is a chief of the Fire Equipment Section in the Fire Research Institute, Tokyo, Japan. He is studying liquid fire properties, water spray properties, rheology of extinguishing agents, and extinction of fires with extinguishing agents.

Fire Studies in Oxygen-Enriched Atmospheres

V. A. Dorr

*Research and Development Department
Ocean Systems, Incorporated
Tarrytown, New York*

(Received January 14, 1970)

ABSTRACT

Studies of the effects of environmental parameters upon combustion in hyperbaric environments and evaluations of selected
materials for flammability in oxygen-enriched atmospheres have
been conducted. Burning rate data for a standard material in oxygen-
nitrogen and oxygen-helium mixtures are presented and a scale of
fire resistance for measuring flammability in oxygen-enriched atmospheres is discussed. Tentative recommendations for some of
the more fire safe materials are included.

INTRODUCTION

The ever-increasing application of oxygen-enriched atmospheres* in hos-
pital hyperbaric chambers, oxygen tents and divers' decompression chambers has pointed up to the vital need for research into the combustion hazards
associated with the use of these environments. Although fires in hyperbaric
and hypobaric chambers are rare, they have occasionally occurred with aston-
ishing suddenness and often fatal results [6, 7, 8, 9]. In order to reduce the
probability of further accidents in oxygen-enriched environments, one must
strive to eliminate any one of the three fundamental prerequisites for a fire:
an ignition source, a fuel and an atmosphere capable of supporting combustion. In practice, it is often difficult or impossible to remove any one of these
requirements with absolute certainty. Attempts should therefore be made to
reduce the contributing effects of all three essential factors, i. e., electrical
items that may serve as potential ignition sources should be avoided, the
quantity of flammable materials in the chamber should be reduced, and the
absolute oxygen concentration and the oxygen partial pressure within the
chamber should be minimized as much as possible.

In order to evaluate the influence of the above factors upon combustion in
oxygen-enriched environments, a study has been conducted to (1) assess the
effects of environmental parameters upon the combustion rate of a standard
material, (2) determine the minimum oxygen concentration required for the
combustion of solid flammables in the presence of nitrogen and helium, and
(3) categorize the flammability hazards of cloth fabrics, elastomers and insula-
tions in hyperbaric environments.

---

* An oxygen-enriched atmosphere (OEA) is generally defined as an atmosphere which contains greater
than 21 mole-% oxygen and/or contains a partial pressure of oxygen greater than 0.21 atmosphere.

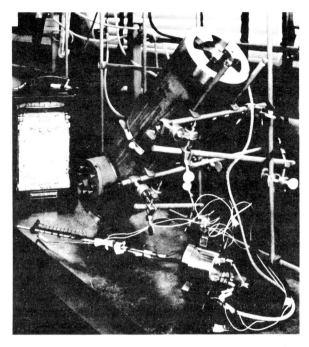

Figure 5. *Fifteen centimeter ID pressure vessel, its closure and sample holder.*

EFFECTS OF ENVIRONMENTAL PARAMETERS UPON COMBUSTION

Small-scale tests and rate determinations are conducted in a 15 cm. ID by 51 cm. long chamber with a working pressure of 40 atm. abs. (Figure 5). A strip of test material is mounted on a series of brass pins and the lower end is held firmly in an igniter grid of chromel wire which may be heated to 1400° F. Thermocouples welded to the igniter wire and mounted on the sample holder allow measurement of ignition temperature and burning rate.

The burning rates of filter paper have been measured in oxygen-nitrogen and oxygen-helium mixtures containing 15% to 100% oxygen over the pressure range of 1 to 10 atm. abs. [3, 4]. Figure 1, a plot of the burning rates of filter paper in oxygen-nitrogen mixtures at an angle of 45° versus the total pressure, shows that the burning rate is accelerated for all gas mixtures as the total pressure is increased. The rate is also accelerated as the oxygen content is increased at any given pressure. In the case of air, 21% oxygen, the combustion rate of filter paper is increased from 1.1 cm./sec. to 2.9 cm./sec. as the pressure is raised from 1 atm. abs. to 10.1 atm. abs. The same material burns at a rate of 2.1 cm./sec. in a 50% oxygen/50% nitrogen mixture at 1 atm. abs., yet this rate decreases to 1.2 cm./sec. as the total pressure is increased to 3.3 atm. abs. by adding nitrogen without changing the oxygen partial pressure of 0.5 atm. The burning rates of filter paper in oxygen-helium mixtures are analogous to the preceding, as seen in Figure 2. The burning rate is accelerated by either an increase in the total pressure of any given gas mixture or an increase in the oxygen concentration at any given total pressure.

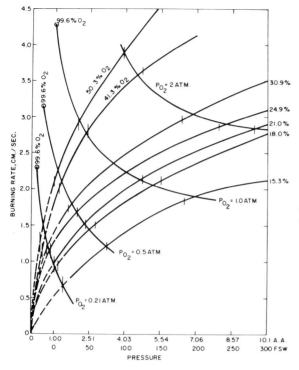

Figure 1. *Burning rates of filter paper at an angle of 45° in oxygen-nitrogen mixtures.*

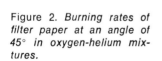

Figure 2. *Burning rates of filter paper at an angle of 45° in oxygen-helium mixtures.*

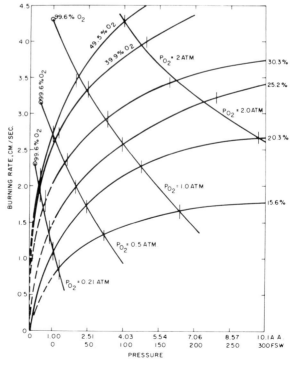

A comparison of the burning rates in helium versus nitrogen (with identical oxygen concentration and total pressure) shows that the combustion process tends to be accelerated in the helium environment. This effect has been observed to be most pronounced at atmospheric pressure in a 30% oxygen atmosphere. In the helium mixture, the burning rate of filter paper at an angle of 45° is measured as 1.9 cm./sec. whereas the burning in the nitrogen mixture is measured as only 1.4 cm./sec., a 26% decrease. The difference in burning rates tends to diminish (in the oxygen concentration range of 15% to 50%) as the total pressure of the mixture is increased. A reduction of the difference in the densities of oxygen-helium and oxygen-nitrogen mixtures at higher pressures probably accounts for this.

MINIMUM OXYGEN CONCENTRATIONS NECESSARY FOR COMBUSTION IN HYPERBARIC ENVIRONMENTS.

The risk of fire is not always increased in hyperbaric environments. At high pressures, the oxygen concentration in a mixture of oxygen and inert gas is normally reduced in order to avoid the danger of oxygen toxicity. This decrease in the oxygen percentage may also render the atmosphere incapable of supporting combustion under certain carefully defined conditions [1, 5]. Three zones representing complete combustion, incomplete combustion and no combustion at all are shown in Figure 3, a plot of oxygen concentration versus total pressure for vertical strips of filter paper in oxygen-nitrogen mixtures. Isobars showing oxygen partial pressures of 0.21 and 1.5 atm. are also shown as these oxygen concentrations represent minimum and maximum partial pressures normally used for a respirable environment in hyperbaric chambers. It is seen that the area denoted ABC lies both within the region of noncombustion and between the two oxygen isobars, thus these conditions will maintain life yet will not support the combustion of ordinarily flammable materials such as paper and cotton cloth. The narcotic effect of nitrogen at high pressure, however, makes its use as a diluent gas unadvisable at partial pressures exceeding approximately 5.5 atm. Therefore, only the area denoted ADE is both physiologically acceptable and free from all risk of accidental fire. The absence of narcosis in oxygen-helium mixtures (up to pressures of at least 35 atm. abs.) produces a much larger and more practical range of gas composition and pressure (Figure 4) that is physiologically satisfactory and still devoid of combustion hazards.

FLAMMABILITY OF MATERIALS IN HYPERBARIC ENVIRONMENTS

When it is impractical to maintain the hyperbaric environment within the region of noncombustion and if all possible sources of ignition within the chamber cannot be precluded with absolute certainty, great care should be exercised in the selection of materials to be placed in the chamber. The results of standard flammability tests in the ambient atmosphere are not valid indications of the burning behavior the same material exhibits under hyperbaric conditions. In our laboratory, we have devised a scale of fire resistance for flammability under oxygen-enriched atmospheric conditions [2, 4, 5]. Materials are tested for combustion in air at atmospheric pressure, compressed air and in oxygen-nitrogen mixtures containing increasing amounts of

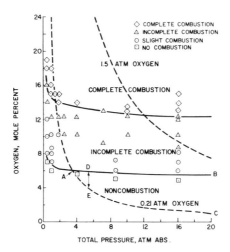

Figure 3. *Three combustion zones for vertical filter paper strips in oxygen-nitrogen mixtures.*

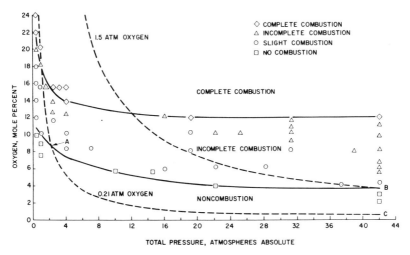

Figure 4. *Three combustion zones for vertical filter paper strips in oxygen-helium mixtures.*

oxygen at a total pressure of one atm. abs. The material is then rated in one of ten classifications described below:

Scale of Fire Resistance

Class 0. Burns readily in air at atmospheric pressure

Class 1. Has an appreciably higher ignition temperature and/or burns at an appreciably lower rate in air at 1 atm abs pressure than cotton cloth or paper. An example of a Class 1 material is wool.

Class 2. Non-flammable or self-extinguishing in air at one atm abs pressure.

Class 3. Self-extinguishing or burns slowly in air at a pressure of 100 feet of sea water (4.03 atm abs).

Class 4. Self-extinguishing or burns slowly in air at a pressure of 200 fsw (7.06 atm abs).

Class 5. Self-extinguishing or burns slowly in a mixture of 25% oxygen and 75% nitrogen at a pressure of 1 atm abs.

Class 6. Self-extinguishing or burns slowly in a mixture of 30% oxygen and 70% nitrogen at a pressure of 1 atm abs.

Class 7. Self-extinguishing or burns slowly in a mixture of 40% oxygen and 60% nitrogen at a pressure of 1 atm abs.

Class 8. Self-extinguishing or burns slowly in a mixture of 50% oxygen and 50% nitrogen at a pressure of 1 atm abs.

Class 9. Non-flammable in 100% oxygen at a pressure of 1 atm abs.

Although over one hundred materials have been tested for flammability and classified [4, 5], there are very few that possess enough intrinsic flame resistance to be considered truly acceptable for use in oxygen-enriched hyperbaric chambers. Test results and comments on several of these materials are presented below.

FABRICS AND CLOTHING

Owens-Corning Beta Fiberglas is a completely nonflammable Class 9 fabric which, perhaps, has the greatest application in oxygen-enriched atmospheres. The material does not burn in pure oxygen at atmospheric pressure even when ignition is attempted with the intense flames of burning cellophane tape. The material does, however, melt under these conditions and small, brittle beads of fused glass remain. The material has very low abrasion resistance (about ⅛ that of nylon) and consequently Beta garments have poor durability. We feel that this is a minor inconvenience in comparison with the greater safety Beta fabric affords over conventional materials. One-piece coveralls made from Beta 4190B (B. Welson Company, Style BW-1027-001) are being used successfully in the Ocean Systems manned diving research currently underway in Tarrytown, N. Y. Another Beta garment, a two-piece suit with parka made from a heavier gauge fabric, is the Fyrepel, Model 320-30-G9.

Although minor skin irritation has been reported in conjunction with the use of glass garments, we have experienced no discomfort when wearing the Welson suit. The abrasion resistance and, presumably, comfort of the fabric may be increased by coating it with Teflon. A sample of the Teflon coated Beta Fiberglas 4190, obtained from B. Welson, was considerably stiffer than the uncoated material. When this was tested in oxygen at atmospheric pressure, the coating did not burn when in contact with the igniter wire alone but when cellophane tape was used to provide a flaming ignition source, the coating burned almost completely off. The DuPont Armalon P.S. 6439 and 63339AS which are also Teflon coated glass fabrics as well as Armalon 98-101 which is Teflon coated Nomex have been rated as Class 7 as the coating burns off in a mixture of 40% oxygen and 60% nitrogen at atmospheric pressure. An additional material obtained from B. Welson, "super Beta", is made by coating the glass fibers with Teflon before weaving and the resultant fabric is strong and more pliable than the coated fabric. The coating did not burn in oxygen even with the flaming ignition source and the material is Class 9. This technique appears to overcome the major limitations of regular Beta Fiberglas but it is still under development and to our knowledge the material is not yet being produced commercially.

Beta may also be obtained in the form of webbing of several different widths from the Carolina Narrow Fabric Company. We have used this material with limited success (due to breakage) for interwoven supports in the bunks and chairs used in our chambers.

There are several other types of fabrics in the Class 8 and Class 9 categories which are currently under development and which may have future application. Ordinary asbestos fabrics contain only about 80% asbestos and 20% of a carrier fabric added for strength. This carrier is usually cotton or a polyester which will burn off intensively in a hyperbaric environment. Uniroyal Fiber and Textile, in their D67504 and D67505 series, has developed a 79% asbestos, 14% Beta Fiberglas and 7% Nomex composite which we rate as Class 9. Although the samples did not burn in oxygen, there were, however, periodic small flashes of light from within the fabric as ignition was attempted. This stems presumably from the interwoven Nomex. The material also is produced with several types of finishes which reduce linting and scuffing of the asbestos. Although the material is rather stiff and heavy for clothing applications, it seems plausible that an adequate, nonflammable blanket (when several layers are sewn in between a cover, e.g. Beta Fiberglas) could be fabricated.

Fiberfrax alumina-silica ceramic fiber from Carborundum is a Class 9 material which is produced as a fabric, felt, board and rope (note that several types must be heat treated at 800°F. for several hours by the customer to remove organic residues before qualifying for Class 9). The material is heavy, coarse and will irritate the skin with prolonged contact. It is a very good insulation material and might also serve as a blanket when placed inside a suitable cover. It might also serve as a good fire blanket to smother fires as it is rated for service up to 2300°F. (this, however, has been shown to be a very ineffective method to extinguish chamber fires [10]). The fiberfrax rope, also nonflammable has a very low tensile strength but this may be increased by using a flexible steel cable in the center.

Several types of inorganic fabrics under development by Union Carbide Corporation have been tested. Zirconia cloth and boron nitride cloth* are Class 9 materials and Thornel carbon fabric is Class 8. Of the three, boron

---

* Boron nitride cloth is also under development by The Carborundum Company.

Table 1. Burning Rates of Mine Safety Appliances Fire Retardant Wool Blanket and Union Carbide Dynel Blanket.

MSA Fire Retardant Wool Blanket No. 04-12487	UCC Dynel Blanket
0.39 cm/sec	0.35 cm/sec
0.45	0.29
0.47	0.28
Average = 0.44[2]	Average = 0.31

1. All samples burned at an angle of 45° in 30% oxygen-70% nitrogen at 15 psia.
2. Wool strips were self-extinguishing in several runs whereas Dynel burned steadily in all runs. Wool, however, always burned with a stronger flame and longer flame front than Dynel.

nitride most closely resembles the weave and appearance of normal cloth. The Carbon Products Division of Union Carbide produces several styles of Ucar electrically conductive cloth in which strands of conductive carbon yarn are woven in a carrier fabric. Style 9966, carbon yarn in E-glass carrier, is Class 8 and style 8020, carbon yarn in B-glass, is Class 5. These fabrics seem particularly well suited for use in heated diving clothing. Two other styles employ cotton and olefin fabrics as the carrier and are readily flammable.

Union Carbide's Dynel fabric, a copolymer of vinyl chloride and acrylonitrile, is a Class 5 material so rated due to its ability to rapidly shrink away from a heat source and therefore prevent ignition. When it does burn, the rate is slow and the heat of combustion appears to be low. Strips of 5 oz./sq. yd. Dynel were burned in 25% oxygen at atmospheric pressure at an angle of 45° and the burning rates were 0.18 and 0.26 cm/sec. In five other attempts, the material was self-extinguishing and rates could not be determined.

Samples of Monsanto Chemical Corporation's X-400 and X-410 fabrics have been supplied to us by the U.S. Navy Clothing and Textile Research Unit. The accompanying technical data sheet from Monsanto describes the X-400 fabric as flameproof in that it "will not burn or produce noxious fumes when subjected to an 1800°F. Meker burner flame." We have verified this statement although it was noted that the fabric initially produced a yellow flame while in contact with the burner flame and the resultant material after this treatment was brittle and would crumble to the touch. In so far as testing these materials in our standard manner, we have rated both the X-400 and X-410 as Class 6. In compressed air at 100 fsw and 200 fsw, both materials smoldered only slightly before self-extinguishing. They also smoldered slightly past the igniter grid in 25% and 30% oxygen at atmospheric pressure but burned completely in 40% oxygen. In addition to possessing improved flame resistance, both materials have the feel and wearability of ordinary textiles and appear to be good candidates for diving clothing as they become more available.

Comparative burning rate tests were conducted on a Mine Safety Appliances fire retardant wool blanket No. 04-12487 and a Union Carbide Dynel blanket and the results are shown in Table 1. MSA informs us that the fire retardant treatment is not resistant to laundering and will wash out in water. Although the burning rate of the wool averaged 0.44 cm/sec versus 0.31 cm/sec for the Dynel, the wool strips were self-extinguishing in several runs whereas the Dynel burned steadily in all runs. Wool, however, always burned with a stronger flame and longer flame front (a nap effect possibly) than Dynel. Of the two blankets, the Dynel appears to be a better choice from a flammability point of view, however, from the same point of view, neither is particularly suited for actual chamber use. Blankets would be safest if custom made in the manner previously described.

An organic material of excellent flame resistance is Pluton heat resistant fabric from the Minnesota Mining and Manufacturing Company (3M). This material appears to be impervious to all ordinary heat sources. When it was exposed to the flame of a natural gas-oxygen torch at ambient conditions, the fabric heated to red hot but cooled upon removal and did not appear to suffer any damage. In a pure oxygen environment, however, the material glowed intensely and disintegrated after contact with the igniter wire. In a mixture of 50% oxygen and 50% nitrogen at atmospheric pressure, the glowing (smoldering) slowly progressed up the strip but was self-extinguishing before the end; Pluton is therefore in Class 8 (style B-1 seems to be slightly more fire resistant than style H-1). To our knowledge, Pluton fabrics have not been used in clothing and bedding applications. The 3M Company states that its susceptibility to damage by abrasion is high and that automatic laundering is not recommended. Otherwise Pluton seems to be a good choice for a compressed air environment from the fire safety point of view.

A new fiber made from polybenzimidazole (commonly referred to as PBI) has been produced by the Celanese Chemical Corporation under contract to the U.S. Air Force. Samples of PBI fabric supplied by the Air Force Materials Laboratory were tested and placed in Class 7. Proposed uses for this material include space capsule parachutes that have to withstand the extreme heat of re-entry and aviation flight suits.

Samples of DuPont's woven brown and white Teflon cloth obtained from Stern and Stern Textiles were basically similar in combustion characteristics under the variety of conditions tested with the exception of pure oxygen at atmospheric pressure in which the white Teflon cloth is significantly less flammable. This difference may be attributed to the approximately 7% carbonaceous residue, formed in the polymerization process, that is left in brown Teflon. The white Teflon has been purified to remove this but is 75% more expensive as a result.

ELASTOMERS

To date, we have located only two nonflammable, Class 9, elastomers. Neither Raybestos-Manhattan's Refset fluoroelastomer nor Thiokol Chemical Corporation's CNR Nitroso Rubber ignites or burns in oxygen at one or two atmospheres absolute pressure. The CNR rubber merely vaporizes in contact with the igniter and the Refset forms a brittle ash. Unfortunately, it appears at this time that Thiokol has discontinued the production of CNR and Raybestos-Manhattan manufactures Refset only as a specialty item.

Other highly nonflammable fluorinated elastomers are currently marketed. While none may be rated as truly nonflammable as the CNR or Refset, they can, however, presently be purchased as regular commercial products. Minnesota Mining and Manufacturing Company's Fluorel brand elastomers are sold to several other companies who complete the processing and sell the finished rubber. One such company, the Mosites Rubber Company has supplied us with samples of Fluorel numbers 1059 and 1071 which we have tested and rated at Class 8. In pure oxygen at one atm abs, the rubber strip burned slowly and completely. A large amount of hydrogen fluoride was apparently released during the combustion as the glass sight port quickly fogged over and was permanently etched. In 50% oxygen-50% nitrogen at one atm abs as well as air at 200 fsw, no sustained burning of the rubber was observed even when the flaming cellophane tape ignition source was utilized.

DuPont's Fairprene 80-080 (Viton), a fluoroelastomer, is a Class 6 material that is not as flame resistant as the Fluorel rubbers discussed previously but is still an improvement over natural rubber. The Fairprene 85-001 (Viton on glass cloth) is only Class 3. The ease of ignition and burning is greater with the thin Viton layer on the coated material than with the thicker, solid slab. Other DuPont elastomers tested such as Fairprene 70-001, Hypalon (Class 3) and straight neoprene (Class 2) are not flame resistant enough for safe use in the chamber.

ELECTRICAL INSULATION

We previously tested a braided copper wire (approximately 1 mm in diameter) insulated with a 7 mil thickness of DuPont's Kapton polyimide film (designated 019-919). The insulation was rated as Class 9 as there was no combustion in 1 atm abs oxygen, however, a Kapton sheet alone is rated as Class 7. It appears that the heat sink effect of the wire plays an important part in the rating of the insulation. One should always take this into consideration when selecting an insulation.

Another flame resistant insulation, tested during the first year, is ITT's Poly/Kynar. Samples of the WTE 1932A (20 gauge) and WTE 1930A (18 gauge) wires were tested and rated as Class 8. Again the heat sink effect of the wire may appear to make the insulation look more nonflammable than it actually is.

We strongly recommend the use of Teflon insulated wire for all chamber wiring. This Class 8 material is commonly being used on wiring for high temperature applications and is readily available on all ordinary sizes and types of wiring. We have used Teflon insulated hook up wiring (Mil-W-16878/D type E, 18 gauge) as leads to the igniter wire and thermocouples during our full scale tests. We have never observed it to sustain combustion during any of the tests although it has flamed and melted off the wire when exposed to direct flames. It is an absolute requirement that additional electrical and mechanical insulation be provided when Teflon insulated wire is used. The abrasion resistance of Teflon is low and the insulation might well wear through when subjected to continuous chafing. The probable cause of the fatal fire in the space environment simulator at Brooks AFB on 31 January 1967 was a short circuit occurring when one of the occupants stepped on an abraded Teflon wire and pressed it against the metal floor [8]. Each Teflon wire should be placed inside a second Teflon or fiberglas sheath and the bundle of doubly insulated wires should be contained inside a flexible metal armor or solid conduit. This scheme should provide ample protection against short circuits and fire.

An excellent choice for all permanent hard wiring in the chamber is General Cable's Mineral Insulated Cable. The conducting wires, imbedded in a mineral insulation, are enclosed in a copper tube. The initial installation effort is greater than for normal wiring due to the care that must be exercised during bending of the cable and sealing of the ends. Moisture penetration may also be a problem and certain techniques have to be employed for its elimination. Once the MI cable is in place, however, it is absolutely noncombustible and virtually impervious to accidental damage.

SUMMARY

Studies of the effects of environmental parameters upon combustion in hyperbaric environments and evaluations of selected materials for flammability in oxygen-enriched atmospheres have been conducted. Test results show that the burning rate of filter paper strips is substantially accelerated as the total pressure of an oxygen-inert gas mixture is increased to pressures to 10 atm abs. Rates are also increased as the oxygen content in the mixture is increased. A comparison of nitrogen and helium as oxygen diluents shows that the combustion process generally proceeds faster in the helium environment, all other factors being equal.

Tentative recommendations for some of the more fire safe materials as well as fabricated end-item products that may have use in hyperbaric chambers are as follows:

Fabrics
    (a) Beta Fiberglas—Owens Corning
    (b) Teflon—DuPont
Elastomers
    (a) Refset—Raybestos—Manhattan
    (b) Fluorel—3M Company
    (c) CNR—Thiokol
Electrical Insulation
    (a) Kapton—DuPont
    (b) Teflon—DuPont
Diver Clothing
    (a) Beta fiberglas coveralls—B. Welson

This work has been supported by Contract N00014-66-CO149 with the Office of Naval Research, Washington, D. C.

REFERENCES

1. G. A. Cook, V. A. Dorr and B. M. Shields, "Region of Noncombustion in Nitrogen-Oxygen and Helium-Oxygen Atmospheres," I and EC Process Design and Development 7, 308 (1968).
2. G. A. Cook, R. E. Meierer and B. M. Shields, "Combustibility Tests on Several Flame-Resistant Fabrics in Compressed Air, Oxygen-Enriched Air, and Pure Oxygen," Textile Research Journal 7, 591 (1967).
3. G. A. Cook, *et al,* "Effects of Gas Composition on Burning Rates Inside Decompression Chambers at Pressures up to 300 Feet of Seawater," Under-Ocean Technology (Proceedings of the 54th Annual Meeting of the Compressed Gas Association, January 17, 1967).

4. G. A. Cook, R. E. Meierer and B. M. Shields, "Screening of Flame-Resistant Materials and Comparison of Helium with Nitrogen for Use in Diving Atmospheres," Defense Documentation Center No. AD-651583 (March 31, 1967).

5. V. A. Dorr and H. R. Schreiner, "Region of Noncombustion, Flammability Limits of Hydrogen-Oxygen Mixtures, Full-Scale Combustion and Extinguishing Tests and Screening of Flame-Resistant Materials," Defense Documentation No. AD-689545 (May 1, 1969).

6. J. V. Harter, "A Review of the Navy Chamber Safety Program" Proceedings of Fire Hazards and Extinguishment Conference, Defense Documentation Center No. AMD-TR-67-2.

7. J. V. Harter, "Fire at High Pressure" Proceedings of the Third Symposium on Underwater Physiology, The Williams and Wilkins Company, Baltimore, 1967.

8. A. G. Swan, "Two Man Space Environment Simulator Accident," Proceedings of Fire Hazards and Extinguishment Conference, Defense Documentation Center No. AMD-TR-67-2.

9. Report of Apollo 204 Review Board to the Administrator, National Aeronautics and Space Administration.

10. L. Segal, *et al*, "Fire Suppression in Hyperbaric Chambers," Fire Journal, May 1966, p. 87.

Victor A. Dorr

Victor A. Dorr is a development chemist in the Research Department of Ocean Systems, Inc. at Tarrytown, New York. He received his B.A. degree in Chemistry from Harpur College of the State University of New York at Binghamton. He worked for Union Carbide Corporation at Tonawanda, New York, before joining Ocean Systems, Inc. in 1968. His experience includes polymer synthesis and development, automotive lubricants, chemical and instrumental analysis, and combustion safety in diving atmospheres.

APPENDIX A

CLASSIFICATION OF MATERIALS ACCORDING TO SCALE OF FIRE RESISTANCE

Class 0

Burns readily in air at atmospheric pressure

Material	Name	Manufacturer
Fabric	Cotton and cotton terrycloth	—
Fabric	Orlon, Style 20543F	Uniroyal
Fabric	Wondershield coated with Fasslon G	J. P. Stevens
Fabric	Ucar Electrically Conductive Fabric Style 9955A (conductive carbon yarn in cotton fabric)	Union Carbide
Fabric	Ucar Electrically Conductive Fabric Style 1103 (conductive carbon yarn in olefin fabric)	Union Carbide
Yarn	Tungsten textile yarn	Union Carbide
Elastomer	Natural Rubber	—
Paint	Heat-resistant aluminum primer	Federal Stock No. 8010-815-2692

Class 1

Has an appreciably higher ignition temperature and/or burns at an appreciably lower rate in air at 1 atm abs pressure than cotton cloth or paper.

Material	Name	Manufacturer
Fabric	Wool	—
Fabric	X-101	Monsanto Chemical
Paint	White cover paint (enamel)	Federal Stock No. 8010-577-4738

Class 2

Nonflammable or self-extinguishing in air at one atm abs pressure.

Material	Name	Manufacturer
Fabric	Roxel [cotton treated with tetrakis (hydroxymethyl) phosphonium chloride (THPC)]	Hooker Chemical
Fabric	Asbeston S/5670	Uniroyal
Fabric	Asbeston S/6555 (asbestos/polyester composite)	Uniroyal
Fabric	Plasticon	Continental Hospital Industries
Fabric	Silastic 2316 coated on 128 glass	Dow Corning
Elastomer	Neoprene	Du Pont
Elastomer	Special Rubber No. 59356	B. F. Goodrich
Elastomer	Silastic S-23416U	Dow Corning
Elastomer	SE-9029 and SE-9044	General Electric
Foam	Experimental urethane foam No. 584RD69	Union Carbide

Class 3

Self-extinguishing or burns slowly in air at a pressure of 100 fsw (4.03 atm abs).

Material	Name	Manufacturer
Fabric	Nomex	Du Pont
Fabric	Fairprene 85-001 (Viton coated fiberglass)	Du Pont
Fabric	Fairprene 72-020 (Hypalon coated nylon)	Du Pont
Fabric	Flameproof Jean cloth	Capital Cubicle
Fabric	Verel V-304	Eastman
Fabric	Brattice cloth	American Brattice Cloth
Fabric	Cotton sateen treated with tris (1-aziridinyl) phosphine oxide (APO)	Dow Chemical
Fabric	50% Nomex/50% THPC treated cotton	Hooker Chemical
Fabric	Green cotton No. 60	Wheeler Protective Apparel
Fabric	Submarine flameproofed mattress cover	Supplied by U. S. Navy Experimental Diving Unit
Elastomer	Fairprene 70-001 (Hypalon)	Du Pont
Felt	Nomex batt	Du Pont

Class 4

Self-extinguishing or burns slowly in air at a pressure of 200 fsw (7.06 atm abs).

Material	Name	Manufacturer
Fabric	Fairprene 5710 (neoprene coated nylon)	Du Pont
Fabric	Fairprene 88-003 (butyl coated Nomex)	Du Pont
Fabric	Dynel	Union Carbide
Fabric	Wool treated with THPC	Hooker Chemical
Fabric	Fire-Retardant Wool Blanket	Mine Safety Appliances
Fabric	Fabric F	David Clark Inc.
Plastic	Hetron 92	Hooker Chemical

Class 5

Self-extinguishing or burns slowly in a mixture of 25% oxygen and 75% nitrogen at a pressure of 1 atm abs.

Material	Name	Manufacturer
Fabric	Silverprened Fiberglass No. 35	Wheeler Protective Apparel
Fabric	Asbeston Cloth (17% flameproof cotton)	Wheeler Protective Apparel
Fabric	Cotton Khaki No. 61	Wheeler Protective Apparel
Fabric	Rovana, patterns 5700, 5800 and 6400	Dow Badische
Fabric	Wondershield	J. P. Stevens
Fabric	Dynel Tent Material	Uniroyal
Fabric	Dynel Blanket	Union Carbide
Fabric	Ucar Electrically Conductive cloth style 8020 (conductive carbon yarn in fiberglass fabric)	Union Carbide
Fabric	CP-2198 (Aluminum coated asbestos)	Johns-Manville
Fabric	Terry Knit Nomex	Du Pont
Fabric	Panel No. 221-158-1 and 2 (hypalon coated fiberglas)	Du Pont
Film	Kapton film type 100H	Du Pont

Class 6

Self-extinguishing or burns slowly in a mixture of 30% oxygen and 70% nitrogen at a pressure of 1 atm abs.

Material	Name	Manufacturer
Fabric	Asbeston S/1445 (asbestos/dynel composite)	Uniroyal
Fabric	Asbeston S/3620-IAR	Uniroyal

Fabric	Navy brattice cloth	American Brattice Cloth
Fabric	X-400	Monsanto Chemical
Fabric	X-410	Monsanto Chemical
Elastomer	Fairprene 80-080 (Viton)	Du Pont

Class 7

Self-extinguishing or burns slowly in a mixture of 40% oxygen and 60% nitrogen at a pressure of 1 atm abs.

Material	Name	Manufacturer
Fabric	PBI (polybenzimidazole)	Celanese Corporation under contract to U. S. Air Force.
Fabric	XF-91 coated fiberglas	Reliable Rubber Products
Fabric	Armalon P.S. 6439 and 63339AS (Teflon coated fiberglass)	Du Pont
Fabric	Armalon 98-101 (Teflon coated Nomex)	Du Pont
Elastomer	XF-91	Reliable Rubber Products
Film	Kapton film types 300H and 200F919	Du Pont

Class 8

Self-extinguishing or burns slowly in a mixture of 50% oxygen and 50% nitrogen at a pressure of 1 atm abs.

Material	Name	Manufacturer
Fabric	Teflon	Du Pont
Fabric	Teflon coated Beta Fiberglas	Supplied by B. Welson
Fabric	Pluton H-1 and B-1	3M
Fabric	Ucar Electrically Conductive Fabric Style 9966 (conductive carbon yarn in fiberglass fabric)	Union Carbide
Fabric	Thornel (carbon fabric)	Union Carbide
Fabric	Avceram CS	FMC
Fabric	100% Rhovyl Knit* (Polyvinylchloride Cloth)	John J. Ryan
Elastomer	Fluorel 1071	Mosites Rubber
Electrical Insulation	Type WTE electric wire insulation	ITT
Plastic	Hetron 92TG + Sb_2O_3	Hooker Chemical

* Conditional classification because the fabric shrinks away from flame and is self-extinguishing. The material is not intrinsically flame resistant.

Class 9

Nonflammable in 100% oxygen at a pressure of 1 atm abs.

Material	Name	Manufacturer
Fabric	Beta Fiberglas	Owens-Corning
Fabric	Beta Fiberglas	Supplied by B. Welson
Fabric	"Super Beta" (Glass fibers coated with Teflon before weaving)	Supplied by B. Welson
Fabric	Boron Nitride Cloth	Union Carbide
Fabric	Zirconia Cloth	Union Carbide
Fabric	D67504 and D67505 series (asbestos/fiberglass composites)	Uniroyal
Fabric, felt, board and rope	Fibergrax Ceramic Fiber (many styles)*	Carborundum
Webbing	Beta Fiberglas webbing	Carolina Narrow Fabrics
Elastomers	CNR Nitroso Rubber	Thiokol
Elastomers	Refset	Raybestos-Manhattan
Paper	Nonflammable Paper (Fiberglass/asbestos composite)	Dynatech
Electrical insulation	Kapton electric wire insulation type 019-919	Du Pont

* Several types must be heat treated (800°F for several hours) to remove organic residues before qualifying for Class 9.

ALICE M. STOLL AND MARIA A. CHIANTA

Naval Air Development Center
Crew Systems Department
Warminster, PA 18974

THERMAL ANALYSIS OF COMBUSTION OF FABRIC IN OXYGEN-ENRICHED ATMOSPHERES*

(Received March 24, 1973)

ABSTRACT: In search of an optimal two-gas space-capsule environment offering minimal hazard from clothing fire, fabric combustion was studied in oxygen-enriched atmospheres of argon, nitrogen, and helium at standard and at hypobaric pressures. From the thermal properties of the gas mixtures used the convective heat transfer coefficient was calculated for each level of pressure and each oxygen concentration. The experimental data showed that at relatively low heating rates, where the effect of the diluent gases could be differentiated from one another, the combustion rate varied inversely with the heat transfer coefficient. At higher heating rates, subtle differences due to specific effects of the diluent gases were over-ridden and destruction rates at each pressure level depended solely upon the mass flow of oxygen, the inert gas serving only to maintain the oxygen concentration. In all instances, the experimental data may be represented by equations of the form $Y = Ce^{nX}$ where Y is the mass flow of oxygen, X is the total heat flow and C and n are constants dependent upon the experimental conditions.

INTRODUCTION

IN STUDIES OF the effect of oxygen-enriched atmospheres on the burning rate of fabrics [1], it was found that destruction rate could be correlated with the mass flow of both oxygen and diluent. It was observed also that pressure level made little difference in destruction rate when the diluent gas was helium while a measurable effect occurred when the denser gases, nitrogen and argon, were the diluents. This too indicated that the retardant effect of the diluent is a function of mass flow, for the absolute difference in mass of helium from one pressure level to another is negligible while the difference in mass of the heavier gases over the same pressure range is considerable. Consequently, no pressure effect was seen with the light gas while a definite effect was seen with the heavy ones.

The correlation of destruction rate with mass flow suggests that both constants, thermal conductivity and specific heat, which depend on mass, may be significant factors in the damping process. Furthermore, it is well known that the thermal conductivity and the time rate of heat capacity (i.e., the product of mass flow and

*Presented in part before the Heat Transfer Division of the American Society of Mechanical Engineers at the Winter Annual Meeting, New York, New York, November 28, 1972.

specific heat) of helium are much greater than that of nitrogen or argon. Both of these circumstances contribute to more rapid removal of heat from the burning site by helium than by argon or nitrogen and therefore should contribute to the observed superior retardation of burning by helium. Thus, the data suggested that investigation of the role of the heat transport properties of the gas media might assist in explaining the mechanism by which the inert gases retard combustion. The present analysis was made for this purpose.

EXPERIMENTAL MATERIALS AND METHOD

The apparatus and experimental method are described in detail in Reference 1. In brief, the apparatus consists of a pressure chamber which encompasses an ignitor coil of nichrome, a stand for holding the fabric specimen, a thermocouple for measuring (approximately) the temperature of the coil and specimen, a flowmeter for measuring precisely the flow of gas into the chamber and appropriate recording and control instruments. Figure 1 shows schematically the chamber (1 cu. ft. in volume); gas tank with regulator valve and flowmeter; altimeter and vacuum adjust valves for setting pressures; specimen mount; heating coil and power supply; and thermocouple for monitoring the ignitor and specimen temperatures.

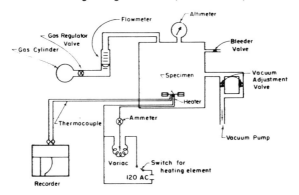

Figure 1. *Pressure chamber with specimen mount.*

The fabric sample was mounted between two square transite plates, 4″ on edge, with a circular central hole 2 5/8″ in diameter. The hole was centered over the ignitor so that the fabric specimen was positioned directly over the ignitor and about 2 mm above it in the early experiments. Later, similar experiments were conducted with the fabric in contact with the ignitor. The fabric used in all experiments was a fire-resistant polyamide, Nomex[1], in a filament fiber, 2/2 twill weave, 3 oz/yd² in weight. It was chosen because its flame-resistant quality so inhibited pyrolysis throughout the entire range of oxygen concentration that distinctive

---

[1] Trade name of E. I. duPont de Nemours textile fiber.

phases in the burning process could be identified more easily in this fabric than in others.

Each specimen was heated to ignition and the heat maintained in the coil until the end of the episode, i.e., throughout burning whether to completion or to self-extinguishment. Three gas mixtures were used, viz., O_2/N_2, O_2/He and O_2/A. Three levels of pressure were used, viz., 14.7, 10.9 and 7.3 psia (equivalent to sea level, 8,000 ft. and 18,000 ft. altitude respectively). At each oxygen concentration the actual flow of oxygen was adjusted for each diluent gas and pressure level to provide the same mass flow of oxygen to the specimen as that delivered at a flow of 15 standard liters/min (SLPM) [1] so that the effects due to each diluent could be separated from those due to oxygen availability alone.

THERMAL PROBLEM, PROCEDURES AND DATA

The objective of the analysis is to determine the heat transport properties of the various gas mixtures as they pertain to the combustion of the fabric.

The total heat input to the system, illustrated in the greatly simplified sketch in Figure 2, is composed of the heat from the ignitor coil, H_h, and the heat generated

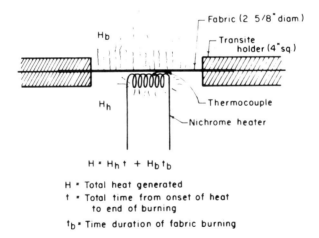

$$H = H_h t + H_b t_b$$

H = Total heat generated
t = Total time from onset of heat to end of burning
t_b = Time duration of fabric burning

Figure 2. *Total heat input.*

by combustion of the fabric, H_b. Since the fabric is not in contact with the coil, it receives heat by radiation and convection as well as hot gas conduction. That part which is supplied by convection is subject to variation as the thermal transport properties of the gas mixtures vary. However, since the gap is small in comparison to the mass of heater coil and fabric involved, these differences may be fairly small and most of the heat may be supplied by radiation. Such considerations do not pertain to the instances in which the fabric was heated by contact with the coil.

In all instances, heat loss proceeds by radiation and convection until the combustion front reaches the holder whereupon conduction heat loss begins to contribute. Since conduction enters only at the end of the burning episode when the burning front of the fabric contacts the holder it may be neglected. Radiation loss, while not insignificant, should be of the same order of magnitude regardless of the gaseous medium since it depends only on the temperature of the fabric as compared with that of the wall. The oxygen content influences the heat flow by the variation it causes in the magnitude and intensity of the combustion reaction, largely a convective process. Thus, of the total heat loss, the greatest variation occurs in the convective portion.

For the analysis of this loss the equation chosen as most nearly approximating the experimental situation is that for the coefficient of heat loss by natural convection from a heated horizontal plate facing upward [2]. This configuration would apply until the fabric burned away whereupon the horizontal plate in that area would be imaginary but the heat generated by the flame front would still be lost as a function of the heat capacity of the gaseous medium. The condition of natural convection was selected as more appropriate than forced convection because the gas flow of 15 SLPM in the relatively large chamber used provided a flow velocity of only 0.088 ft/sec across the specimen. The actual flow required to maintain 15 SLPM as the pressure was reduced, increased to about 20 L/min at 10.9 psia and 30 L/min at 7.3 psia, a velocity of 0.132 and 0.176 ft/sec respectively, or essentially quiet air as determined in conditioned chambers maintained at fixed temperatures [3]. The analysis, however, is complicated by the fact that after the fabric ignites, the gas flow changes from laminar to turbulent as burning progresses. Also, this change occurs at different times after ignition depending on the burning rate. However, the difference effected in the equation (Equation 1 below) is confined to the constant, C, and the exponent, x, which depend upon the particular situation and which are adjusted to adapt to the appropriate flow type:

$$\frac{h_c L}{k_f} = C \left[\frac{L^3 \rho_f^2 \, g \, \beta_f \, \Delta t}{\mu_f^2} \left(\frac{c_p u}{k} \right)_f \right]^x \tag{1}$$

where

h_c = heat loss by convection, coef., Btu/hr ft^2 °F

L   = length in feet

k_f = thermal conductivity at t_f, Btu/hr ft^2 °F/ft

t_f = "film" temperature = $(t_s + t_a)/2$, t_s for surface, t_a for ambient

C   = constant determined by particular situation

ρ_f = density at t_f, lb/ft^3

g   = acceleration due to gravity, 4.17×10^8 ft/hr^2

β_f = coef. of volumetric expansion, reciprocal °F

Δt = temperature difference (fabric − gas)

c_p = specific heat, Btu/lb °F

μ = viscosity, lb/hr ft = 2.42x centipoises

x   = exponent determined by situation

The data required to insert in this equation were derived from a variety of sources and calculated to yield the information in appropriate units.

The specific heat of each gas mixture is determined from Equation 2 [4] :

where:

$$c_{pm} = w\,c_{p1} + (1-w)c_{p2}$$

c_{pm} = specific heat of mixture

$$w = \text{mass fraction of component 1} = \frac{m_1}{m_1 + m_2}$$

$$\text{where } m_1 = \text{weight of gas \#1, etc.} \tag{2}$$

and as cited in [5] :

$$w = \frac{(\%D \times MWD)}{(\%\,O_2 \times MWO_2) + (\%D \times MWD)} \tag{3}$$

where

D   = diluent gas = component #1

MW   = molecular weight

The viscosity of the binary mixtures is calculated according to the method of C. R. Wilke [6] cited in [4] :

$$\mu_m = \frac{\mu_1}{1 + (x_2/x_1)\,(\phi_{12})} + \frac{\mu_2}{1 + (x_1/x_2)\,(\phi_{21})} \tag{4}$$

where

$$\phi_{ij} = \frac{[1 + (\mu_i/\mu_j)^{1/2}\,(M_i/M_j)^{1/4}]^2}{\cdot(4/\sqrt{2})\,[1 + (M_i/M_j)]^{1/2}}$$

where

$M_i + M_j$ = molecular weights of the pure gases

$x_1 + x_2$ = mole fractions

$\mu_i + \mu_j$ = viscosities of pure components

Thermal conductivity of the binary mixture is found by the method of Lindsay and Bromley [7] cited in [4] :

$$k_m = \frac{k_1}{1 + A_1 \, (x_2/x_1)} + \frac{k_2}{1 + A_2 \, (x_1/x_2)} \tag{5}$$

where

k_m = thermal conductivity of the mixture, other symbols are defined as in Equation 4 above, and A_1 and A_2 are Wassiljewa constants [8] as cited in [4]. These are:

$$A_1 = 1/4 \left\{ 1 + \left[\frac{\mu_1}{\mu_2} \left(\frac{M_2}{M_1} \right)^{\frac{3}{4}} \frac{1 + (S_1/T)}{1 + (S_2/T)} \right]^{\frac{1}{2}} \right\}^2 \frac{1 + (S_{12}/T)}{1 + (S_1/T)}$$

$$A_2 = 1/4 \left\{ 1 + \left[\frac{\mu_2}{\mu_1} \left(\frac{M_1}{M_2} \right)^{\frac{3}{4}} \frac{1 + (S_2/T)}{1 + (S_1/T)} \right]^{\frac{1}{2}} \right\}^2 \frac{1 + (S_{12}/T)}{1 + (S_2/T)}$$

where

T = absolute temperature, $^\circ$K
S = Sutherland constant

and

$$S_{12} = \sqrt{S_1 \cdot S_2}$$

The density of the gas mixtures varies in proportion to their percentage composition. Therefore,

$$\rho_{O_2 D} = x \, (\rho_{O_2}) + (1-x) \, \rho_D \tag{6}$$

where

$\rho_{O_2 D}$ = density of oxygen mixture at given temperature and pressure

x = percentage of O_2 present

ρ_D = density of diluent at given temperature and pressure

and

ρ_{O_2} = density of oxygen at same temperature and pressure

Table 1 presents the properties of the pure gases of interest at 80°F as compiled from various engineering handbooks and the data book of the supplier of the gases

56

used [9]. Units are chosen to provide dimensionless numbers in accordance with McAdams' usage [2, pp. 135, 180].

Table 1. Properties of Pure Gases at 80° F and 14.7 psia

Gas	Density lb/ft³	Sp. Heat Btu/lb °F	Viscosity(u) lb/hr ft	Conductivity Btu/hr ft°F	Diffusivity ft²/hr	Prandtl *
Helium	0.1106	1.2420	0.0488	0.08640	6.2900	0.702
Oxygen	0.0812	0.2198	0.0499	0.01546	0.8662	0.709
Nitrogen	0.0713	0.2486	0.0432	0.01514	0.8542	0.713
Argon	0.1016	0.1252	0.0541	0.01030	0.8097	0.658

These data were used in a computer program to solve for h_c, the heat transfer coefficient. The value of 1200°F, calculated from the approximate temperature of the flaming fabric (∿ 1290°F as measured by thermocouple) was used for Δt, the temperature difference between the fabric and the gas. The values for C, the constant, and x, the exponent, were determined within the program on the basis of the form of the curve,

$$Y = CX^n \text{ where}$$

$$Y = \frac{h_c L}{k_f}; X = \frac{L^3 \rho^2 g^{\beta} f^{\Delta} t}{\mu^2} \left(\frac{c_p \mu}{k}\right)_f, \text{ and } n = x$$

Thus, when turbulent flow was indicated by values of X from 2×10^7 to 3×10^{10}, C became 0.14 and n = 1/3. Similarly, in the laminar range, X from 10^5 to 2×10^7, C = 0.54 and n = 1/4 [2]. The resultant data and the constants used in the computations at 14.7 psia are shown in Table 2 for mixtures ranging from pure oxygen to pure diluent in 10% decrements of O_2.

(It is noteworthy that under these conditions the heat transfer coefficient of pure helium is only 1.7 times that of pure oxygen even though its thermal conductivity is almost 6 times as great. At the 50–50 point O_2/He is only 1.3 times as effective as O_2/N_2 as a heat loss medium while argon and its mixtures exhibit even less heat transport capacity than oxygen alone. Furthermore, the relative magnitudes of these values may be expected to pertain in similar heat loss situations irrespective of the dimensions of the surface because they reflect the characteristics of the gaseous media themselves.)

Additional solutions appropriate to the other two levels of pressure were also carried out. The specific heat, thermal conductivity and viscosity depend upon pressure only in the vicinity of the critical point defined for each gas in Table 3.

57

Table 2. Heat Transfer Coefficients of Gas Mixtures * †

Gas Mixture Mole Fraction O_2	Argon	Conductivity Btu/hr ft°F	Density lb/ft^3	Specific Heat Btu/lb °F	Viscosity lb/hr ft	Heat Transfer Coefficient Btu/hr ft^2 °F
1.00	0	0.01546	0.08120	0.21980	0.04990	4.92066
0.90	0.10	0.01492	0.08324	0.20828	0.05038	4.78337
0.80	0.20	0.01439	0.08528	0.19730	0.05084	4.64640
0.70	0.30	0.01386	0.08732	0.18683	0.05129	4.50740
0.60	0.40	0.01334	0.08936	0.17683	0.05173	4.36859
0.50	0.50	0.01282	0.09140	0.16728	0.05215	4.22821
0.40	0.60	0.01231	0.09344	0.15813	0.05256	4.08806
0.30	0.70	0.01180	0.09548	0.14938	0.05297	3.94597
0.20	0.80	0.01129	0.09752	0.14099	0.05335	3.80260
0.10	0.90	0.01079	0.09956	0.13293	0.05373	3.65940
0	1.00	0.01030	0.10160	0.12520	0.05410	3.51690

O_2 Helium

1.00	0	0.01546	0.08120	0.21980	0.04990	4.92066
0.90	0.10	0.01842	0.07419	0.23381	0.05047	5.29546
0.80	0.20	0.02179	0.06717	0.25080	0.05106	5.65251
0.70	0.30	0.02567	0.06015	0.27181	0.05167	5.99313
0.60	0.40	0.03018	0.05315	0.29849	0.05227	6.31798
0.50	0.50	0.03548	0.04613	0.33345	0.05783	6.42403
0.40	0.60	0.04180	0.03912	0.38130	0.05238	6.66725
0.30	0.70	0.04945	0.03210	0.45075	0.05350	7.10579
0.20	0.80	0.05890	0.02509	0.56070	0.05326	7.57284
0.10	0.90	0.07073	0.01807	0.76116	0.05206	8.00321
0	1.00	0.08640	0.01106	1.24200	0.04880	8.35657

O_2 Nitrogen

1.00	0	0.01546	0.08120	0.21980	0.04990	4.92066
0.90	0.10	0.01540	0.08021	0.22235	0.04923	4.90877
0.80	0.20	0.01534	0.07922	0.22497	0.04856	4.89695
0.70	0.30	0.01528	0.07823	0.22766	0.04790	4.88486
0.60	0.40	0.01523	0.07724	0.23041	0.04723	4.87410
0.50	0.50	0.01517	0.07625	0.23324	0.04656	4.86352
0.40	0.60	0.01511	0.07526	0.23615	0.04589	4.85191
0.30	0.70	0.01505	0.07427	0.23914	0.04522	4.84036
0.20	0.80	0.01499	0.07328	0.24220	0.04454	4.82914
0.10	0.90	0.01493	0.07229	0.24536	0.04387	4.81772
0	1.00	0.01488	0.07130	0.24860	0.04320	4.80520

*Figures obtained from handbooks and computer; significance of heat transfer coefficient no better than third decimal place.

†L = 0.219 ft   P = 14.7 psia t_a = 80°F

Table 3. *Critical Point, Pressure and Density of Pure Gases*

Gas	Temp (°C)	Pressure (atm)	Density (gm/cm³)
Argon	−1.22	48.0	0.531
Helium	−267.9	2.3	0.0693
Nitrogen	−147.1	33.5	0.3110
Oxygen	−118.8	49.7	0.430

The conditions of the present study are far from the critical point of any of the gases, therefore no changes were needed in these values. Density is directly proportional to the pressure so that ρ is easily found at each of the new pressure levels as $\rho = p^1/p_{atm} \times \rho_{atm}$ where p^1 is the new pressure, p_{atm} is atmospheric pressure, and ρ_{atm}, the density at atmospheric pressure. These data were used in the same computer program and the heat transfer coefficient found for the levels of 10.9 and 7.3 psia. All values for h_c at the three levels of pressure are shown in Figure 3,

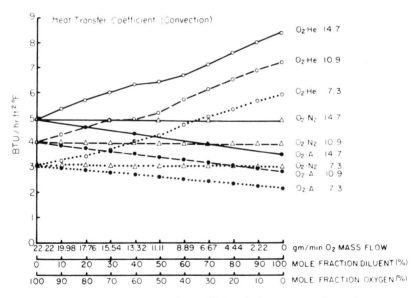

Figure 3. *Convective heat transfer coefficient (h_c) versus mass flow of oxygen.*

correlated with the mass flow of oxygen in gm/min at the mixture flow rate of 15 SLPM. A change in slope occurs in each O_2/He curve at the zone of transition from laminar flow (at the lower O_2 levels) to turbulent; in all other instances the curves are constant in slope and the flow is turbulent.

The total heat generated in the system (H, Figure 2) during any burning episode is the sum of the heat supplied by the heater coil (H_h) and the heat resulting from combustion of the fabric (H_b) multiplied by the burning time. The first term, H_h, may be found from the resistance of the nichrome coil, the measured current or voltage and the burning time:

$$H_h = R\,i^2\ t \text{ or } E\,i\,t$$

where

$$
\begin{aligned}
R &= \text{resistance of the coil} &&= 2.06\Omega \\
i &= \text{current} &&= 9.6 \text{ amp} \\
E &= \text{voltage} &&= 20 \text{ volts}
\end{aligned}
$$

and

$$t = \text{time.}$$

The second term, H_b, may be determined by DuLong's Rule or Mahler's Rule [10], both of which are based on the caloric value of each chemical element in the material being burned in proportion to its presence in the molecule:

DuLong's Formula:

$$H_b = 14,650C + 62,100H - 5,400(O + N)$$

Mahler's Formula:

$$H_b = 14,650C + 62,100H(H - 1/8\ O)$$

(present material completely composed of C,H,O and N).

In the present experiments H_h was 192 watts or 45.9 cal/sec and H_b, 11,735 Btu/lb or 6.54 cal/mg. If the heat of combustion greatly exceeds the coil heat, then the latter could be neglected. However, at 6.54 cal/mg a burning rate of about 7 mg/sec produces enough heat to equal that supplied by the coil. Therefore, in assessing the influence of heat transport on burning rate at given oxygen flows, it is necessary to consider the entire heat produced rather than only that due to combustion. The total heat generated, H, may be determined as:

$$H = H_h\,t + H_b\,t_b \tag{7}$$

where

t = total time from onset of heat to end of burning and t_b = time duration of fabric burning, i.e., from ignition to completion or extinction.

Then the total heat flow may be calculated as the coil heat supply rate, 45.9 cal/sec, plus the observed burning rate in mg/sec times 6.54 cal/mg, the heat of combustion of the fabric.

RESULTS AND DISCUSSION

In the instance of heat supplied without contact between the coil and the fabric, the correlations shown in Figure 4 were obtained. Here it is seen that the log of the mass flow of oxygen (ordinate) is directly related to the total heat flow. At each pressure level the curves representative of the three O_2 diluent mixtures converge on the same point at the maximum O_2 flow rate (100%). At concentrations less than 100% O_2, the curves diverge in a manner commensurate with the differences in heat transfer coefficient (Figure 3), i.e., the higher the coefficient at a given O_2 level, the lower the heat flow and (since the coil input remains constant) the slower the burning rate. At increasingly low pressures the burning rates are proportionately slower. However, the heat transfer coefficients at these pressures are also lower, therefore, this trend is in the direction opposite to that expected if heat transport capacity alone were to account for control of the burning rate at any given O_2 mass flow. Furthermore, if heat transport capacity were the sole controlling factor, at points of equal heat coefficients and equal O_2 mass flow, the same destruction rates would be observed irrespective of gas composition. The data in Table 4 show that the rates at these points (located graphically as the crossover points in Figure 3) are not the same. Instead, there is a difference between rates in different gas mixtures at the same pressure level differences (e.g., O_2/A at 14.7 psia and O_2/He at 10.9 psia = a difference of 1.5 mg/sec; O_2/N_2 at 14.7 and O_2/He at 10.9 = 2.1) and in the same gas mixtures at different pressure level differences (e.g., O_2/A at 10.9 and O_2/He at 7.3 = 1.3; O_2/A at 14.7 and O_2/He at 7.3 = 5.9).

In contrast, the experimental data obtained from heating the specimen by contact with the ignitor, at approximately the same heat output of the coil, reveal no effect due to the nature of the diluent gas. As seen in Figure 5, at each pressure level, all the data points cluster about the same line to yield three parallel curves for the three pressure levels. In this situation, differences in total heat flow attributable to specific effects of the diluent gas are obliterated and the burning rate depends entirely on the oxygen concentration and the pressure level. Tabulating the destruction rate data at equivalent heat coefficient and oxygen flow rates as before now

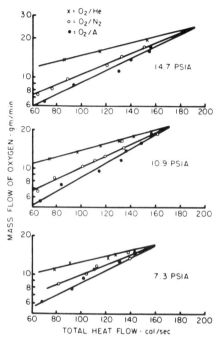

Figure 4. *Oxygen mass flow vs. total heat flow (no contact) at three pressure levels.*

Table 4. Comparison of Destruction Rates of Fabric in Different Gas Mixtures at Points of Equal Oxygen Mass Flow Rates and Equal Heat Transfer Coefficient Values

O_2 Flow gm/min	Heat Transfer Coefficient (h_c) BTU/hr ft^2 °F	Gas at psia		Dest. Rate mg/sec		Difference mg/sec
		#1	#2	#1	#2	(#1 - #2)
17.76	4.6	O_2/A 14.7	O_2/He 10.9	17.0	15.5	1.5
15.76	4.9	O_2/N_2 14.7	O_2/He 10.9	14.4	12.3	2.1
15.76	3.7	O_2/A 10.9	O_2/He 7.3	16.1	14.8	1.3
13.76	4.0	O_2/N_2 10.9	O_2/He 7.3	12.9	11.1	1.8
11.55	4.2	O_2/A 14.7	O_2/He 7.3	10.9	5.0	5.9
7.87	4.8	O_2/N_2 14.7	O_2/He 7.3	3.6	*	-
6.77	3.9	O_2/A 14.7	O_2/N_2 10.9	4.6	2.8	1.8
3.33	3.3	O_2/A 10.9	O_2/N_2 7.3	Off scale		

*Did not burn.

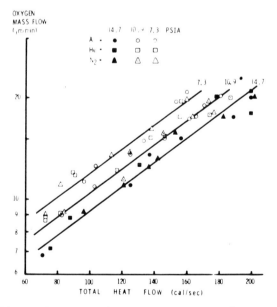

Figure 5. Oxygen mass flow versus total heat flow (specimen in contact with heating coil) at three pressure levels.

discloses an orderly difference of about 2 mg/sec between points at 14.7 psia and 10.9 psia and about double this difference between 14.7 and 7.3 psia where the pressure level difference is about double (Table 5). It is possible that the difference due to pressure level may be attributed to chemical kinetics. However, it is also possible that it shows up because the equation used for calculating heat transport capacity applies to natural convection rather than forced convection and the actual flow, however small, does double and triple at the lower pressures. The latter possibility can be explored by using the equation for forced convection but this has not been done yet. It is likely that the differences attributable specifically to the nature of the diluent gases are obscured by the greater heating rate effected by contact of the fabric with the heating coil. This point could be resolved experimentally by removing the coil after ignition of the specimen occurs. However, the whole effect is so weak there is little practical worth in expending the time and resources required to generate these data. Of more importance is the fact that in the face of relatively vigorous heating the efficacy of the inert gas in slowing combustion is based simply on its efficiency as a diluent for the oxygen present. This effect is illustrated in Figure 6 where the destruction rate is correlated with mass flow of diluent. The curves are superimposable so that all data may be represented by the same curves by displacing the destruction rate on the abscissa approximately 2 mg/sec to the right for each decrement of approximately 4 psia in pressure. Now it is seen that the same extent of limitation may be achieved with less than 2 gm/min of He as is obtained with more than 10 gm/min of N_2 or 16 gm/min of A.

COMMENT

The original observations relating destruction rate to the fire-retardant aspects of the gas mixtures are discussed in detail in Reference 11. For the present purpose, the analysis of the thermal aspects of the burning process, it is pertinent to note that the general form of the combustion process may be deduced from the experimental data. As seen in Figure 3, there is a direct and linear relationship (except in the transition zone between laminar and turbulent flow) between the heat transfer coefficient and the mass flow of oxygen. Then, since the total heat flow involved in the combustion process is related directly to the log of the mass flow of oxygen (Figures 4 and 5), the main controlling factor in the burning process, it follows that the combustion process itself may be expressed by equations of general form $Y = CX^n$ which is the form of Equation 1.

Furthermore, the coefficient for mass transfer with respect to the gaseous media is entirely analogous to that for heat transfer [4]. Therefore, the experimental data should bear the same relationship to mass transfer as to heat transfer. In the instance of mass transfer, $Y = h_D L/D$, the dimensionless mass transfer coefficient, analogous to $h_c L/k$, and $X = f (Gr_D, Sc)$, the Grashof number for mass transfer, and the Schmidt number for molecular diffusivity, respectively, analogous to the Grashof and Prandtl numbers in heat transfer. Of course, these relationships are speculative and far from all-inclusive.

Table 5. Comparison of Destruction Rates of Fabric in Different Gas Mixtures at Points of Equal Heat Transfer Coefficient Values, Fabric in Contact with Ignitor

O_2 Flow gm/min	Heat Transfer Coefficient (h_c) BTU/hr ft^2 °F	Gas at psia		Dest. Rate mg/sec		Difference mg/sec (#1 - #2)
		#1	#2	#1	#2	
17.76	4.6	O_2/A 14.7	O_2/He 10.9	20.2	17.9	2.3
15.76	4.9	O_2/N_2 14.7	O_2/He 10.9	19.2	16.9	2.3
15.76	3.7	O_2/A 10.9	O_2/He 7.3	16.0	13.8	2.2
13.76	4.0	O_2/N_2 10.9	O_2/He 7.3	15.8	13.6	2.2
11.55	4.2	O_2/ A 14.7	O_2/He 7.3	12.9	8.8	4.1
7.87	4.8	O_2/N_2 14.7	O_2/He 7.3	6.2	2.1	4.1

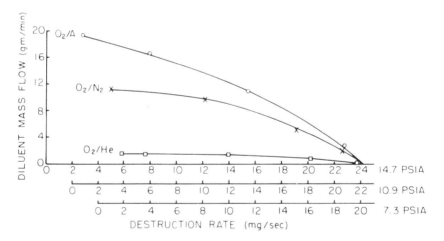

Figure 6. *Mass flow of diluent gases versus destruction rate of fabric.*

Reaction rate theory, too, must have a bearing on the total analysis, for all these mechanisms enter into the combustion process at one stage or another. Indeed, a complete understanding of the broad relationship demonstrated here undoubtedly involves a simultaneous consideration of combinations of all these processes, a formidable task. In the meantime, it is of considerable practical value to be able to express quite accurately for a given combustion situation the effect of variation in composition and pressure of the gaseous medium by use of equations of this familiar general form.

CONCLUSION

It is concluded from the present analysis that flame propagation under the conditions of essentially quiet air flow depends primarily upon the oxygen mass flow available to the specimen. When heating of the specimen is accomplished at a slow rate as in the instance of no contact between ignitor and fabric, differences in damping ability of the three inert gases can be discerned and related to the differences in heat transport capacity of the mixtures. When heating is more intense, as during contact with the ignitor, these differences are obliterated.

It is concluded, further, that whether the heat transport of the gaseous medium or the mass transport on combustion of the material is considered to be the dominant influence, the experimental data fit an equation of the general form $Y = Ce^{nX}$ where Y is the mass flow of oxygen; C and n, constants appropriate to the experimental conditions; and X, the destruction rate or a function thereof (such as heat flow). This observation is of considerable practical importance because it provides a means of predicting from only two or three isolated empirical data points the effect of oxygen dilution by inert gases throughout an entire range of combustion.

REFERENCES

1. M. A. Chianta and A. M. Stoll, "Effect of Inert Gases on Fabric Burning Rate," Aerospace Med. 40: #12, Dec. 1969, pp. 1304–1306.
2. W. H. McAdams, Heat Transmission, 3rd ed., McGraw-Hill Book Co., Inc., New York, Toronto and London, 1954, p. 180.
3. A. P. Gagge, "Standard Operative Temperature," *Temperature: Its Measurement and Control in Science and Industry*, Reinhold Publishing Corp., New York, N.Y., 1941, p. 550.
4. R. G. Eckert and Robert M. Drake, Jr., *Heat and Mass Transfer*, McGraw-Hill Book Co., Inc., New York, 1959, p. 494.
5. Ibid., p. 440.
6. C. R. Wilke, *J. Chem. Physics* 8: 517, 1950.
7. A. L. Lindsay and L. A. Bromley, *Ind. Eng. Chem.* 42: 1, 508, 1950.
8. A. Wassiljewa, *Physik Z.*, 5: 737, 1904.
9. *Matheson Gas Data Book*, 4th Ed., The Matheson Co., Inc., East Rutherford, N.J., 1966.
10. *Scott's Standard Methods of Chemical Analysis*, N. H. Furman, Ed., 5th Ed. Vol. I, D. Van Nostrand Co., Inc., Princeton, N.J., New York, Toronto and London, Mar. 1958, p. 1187.
11. M. A. Chianta and A. M. Stoll, "Fire Retardance of Mixtures of Inert Gases and Oxygen," Aerospace Med. 44: #2, Feb. 1973, pp. 169–173.

A. M. Stoll

Alice M. Stoll, Head of the Biophysics Laboratory, Crew Systems Department, Naval Air Development Center. Background in the biophysics and physiology of burns and biotechnology of heat transfer. Interest in present work derived from accidental burning of experimental subjects in simulated space capsule clothing fire which occasioned a study of O_2-enrichment effects on fabric flammability. Heat transfer analysis was made on experimental data obtained in this investigation.

M. A. Chianta

Maria A. Chianta, Research Chemist in Biophysics Laboratory, Crew Systems Department, Naval Air Development Center, responsible for conduct of study of O_2-enriched atmospheres of inert gases suitable for space capsule environment offering life support with minimal fire hazard. Data in present report was generated during the phase of study dealing with fabric flammability and subjected to heat transfer analysis as part of an effort to determine the damping mechanism of various gas mixtures.

AUTHORS' NOTE

Opinions and conclusions contained in this report are those of the authors. They are not to be construed as necessarily reflecting the views or endorsement of the Department of the Navy.

W. J. PARKER[1]

Fire Research Section
Building Research Division, IAT
National Bureau of Standards

FLAME SPREAD MODEL FOR CELLULOSIC MATERIALS*

(Received May 11, 1972)

ABSTRACT: Downward flame spread along a white index card has been investigated in some detail. Visual observations as well as temperature measurements confirm the release of the pyrolysis gases underneath the flame rather than ahead of it. The extension of the flame beyond the pyrolysis zone due to gaseous diffusion preheats the surface to the pyrolysis temperature by gas phase heat conduction thus causing the flame to move. Because of symmetry the downward flame spread on each side of the card can be treated as flame propagation along a single surface. A flame spread burner was constructed to simulate this surface. An equation was developed to predict the flame spread rate.

INTRODUCTION

IN SPITE OF THE long history of serious fires involving cellulosic materials, no adequate theory of flame spread along them yet exists. In order to establish such a theory, the simplest possible flame spread case should be singled out for extensive study. In this research the downward spread of flame along an oven dried 3 X 5 inch white unruled index card was investigated in a quiescent atmosphere. These cards are in infinite supply, have a negligible cost, represent a typical cellulosic material, and are thin enough to prevent large temperature differences through the thickness of the sample. The cards were mounted vertically so that the flames on both sides were symmetrical. The burning card could then be resolved into two burning surfaces back to back. The concept of a single surface makes it possible to model the flame spread with the artificial flame spread burner described below. Downward flame spread was chosen because it is slow enough to follow visually.

There is a popular belief that a flame moves along a cellulosic material by propagating into a combustible mixture of air and pyrolysis gases distilled from the surface ahead of the flame front [1]. Usually it is assumed that this surface is heated to the pyrolysis temperature by radiative and convective heat transfer. How-

*This work was performed at the Naval Radiological Defence Laboratory as part of a project supported by the Defense Atomic Support Agency and was originally presented at the 1969 Meeting of the Central States Section of The Combustion Institute Held at the University of Minnesota in March 1969.
[1] Formerly Naval Radiological Defense Laboratory, San Francisco, California 94135

ever, these processes appear inadequate when it is considered that (1) convective air flow is toward the flame, and (2) the radiation level outside of a small flame from burning cellulose is extremely low. Solid phase heat conduction does not seem to be an important contributor either since a flame will propagate across a 1 mm gap in the card with no decrease in flame spread rate.

VISUAL OBSERVATIONS

Visual observations of the flame spread suggest that the pyrolysis gases are released entirely behind rather than in front of the flame front. This can be seen most readily by watching the progress of the flame moving down the white card in a darkened room. The pyrolysis zone is clearly visible under the flame as a black charring region bordered by a very thin brownish band indicating the onset of pyrolysis. The lower edge of the flame is defined by the bottom edge of the luminous blue band which is caused by the reflection of the flame from the uncharred white card underneath. The upper edge of the band marks the beginning of the charring region where the reflection from the underlying surface vanishes. This can be seen in Figure 1, although it is more graphic to simply ignite the top of a white card in the dark and watch it. The brighter region at the top is where the char is being consumed by glowing. The bright regions at the edge and along the tips in the card is due to an accentuation of the glowing. In other areas the

Figure 1. *Flame progressing down a white index card in a darkened room (front view).*

enhanced brightness is due to a higher luminosity yellow flame caused by a local increase in the richness of the fuel air mixture. If a mark is placed on the card and the flame is suddenly blown out at the instant it passes over the mark, no deterioration of the card is in evidence within 1.3 mm of the mark. The flame zone appears to start slightly more than 1.3 mm below the pyrolysis zone and to extend about

1.3 cm above it. The downward extension of the flame is due to diffusion of the pyrolysis vapors.

The downward flame spread rate in a quiescent atmosphere was observed visually to be 0.148 cm/s (3.5 in/min) for cards dried for an hour in a vacuum oven at 100°C.

A PROPOSED FLAME SPREAD MECHANISM

An idealized sketch of the flame traveling down the card is shown in Figure 2. The dashed curve shows the limits of the flame heated gases. The extension of the flame and this hot gas zone below the pyrolysis zone preheats the surface

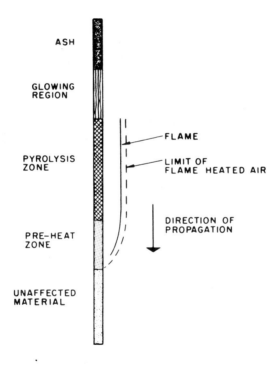

Figure 2. *Idealization of flame spread down the white index card.*

principally by gas phase heat conduction. As the surface temperature is raised to that of active pyrolysis in the neighborhood of 300°C, the pyrolysis zone moves down causing the flame to progress at a rate

$$V = \epsilon/t_p \qquad (1)$$

where ϵ is the length of the preheat zone and t_p is the time required to heat the surface to the pyrolysis temperature, T_p. This time is given by

$$t_p = (\rho cz/2)\,(T_p - T_o)\,/\,q \tag{2}$$

where ρ is the density of the material, c is its heat capacity, z is its thickness, T_p is the threshold temperature of active pyrolysis, T_o is the ambient temperature, and q is the net rate of heat transfer per unit area to each surface.

Assuming that the heat transfer to the surface is by gas phase heat conduction while the heat loss is due primarily to thermal radiation from the solid surface which can be considered to have an emissivity of unity, the net heat transfer is given by

$$q = \lambda\,\frac{\partial T}{\partial x} - \sigma(T^4 - T_o^{\,4}) \tag{3}$$

where λ is the thermal conductivity of the gas at the surface temperature which varies between T_o and T_p, $\frac{\partial T}{\partial x}$ is the normal temperature gradient in the gas at the surface, and σ is the Stefan Boltzmann constant. According to Equation 3, one might expect q to vary through the heating period so that an effective value of q would have to be determined. However, as will be seen later, q appears to be remarkably constant over the preheating period at least for the index cards used for this experiment.

By combining Equations 1, 2 and 3 we can obtain an overall formula for the flame spread velocity,

$$V = 2\,\epsilon\,(\lambda\,\frac{\partial T}{\partial x} - \sigma\,(T^4 - T_o^{\,4}\,))\,/\,\rho cz\,(T_p - T_o). \tag{4}$$

To a very crude approximation neglecting heat absorption in the gases and the change in thermal conductivity with temperature

$$\frac{\partial T}{\partial x} \approx (T_f - T_o)\,/\,d \tag{5}$$

Where T_f is the flame temperature at the lowest point on the card and d is the flame standoff distance there. Since the surface temperature is still low at this point, we let $\sigma\,(T^4 - T_o^{\,4}) = 0$. Combining Equations 4 and 5, we get

$$V = 2\,\epsilon\,\lambda\,(T_f - T_o)\,/\,\rho czd\,(T_p - T_o) \tag{6}$$

Although, in principle, we should be able to calculate ϵ and d, this has not been done in this paper. Those parameters have had to be measured. Before proceeding on to a justification of the proposed model, the flame spread velocity will be estimated by means of Equation 6 using the following values for the parameters: $\epsilon \approx 1.5$ mm (width of flame extension as measured on Figure 1 and confirmed by visual observations of the flame), $d \approx 1$ mm (visual observations of the flame standoff distance at the leading edge of the flame), $\lambda \approx 2.5 \times 10^{-4}$ W/(cm deg) (thermal conductivity of air at ambient temperature [2]), $T_f \approx 1500°C$ (temperature at beginning of the luminous zone of an 8.70% natural gas in air flame from Lewis and Von Elbe [3]), $T_p \approx 280°C$ (threshold of active pyrolysis as observed in the thermogravametric curves of Tang and Neil [4]), $T_0 = 20°C$, $\rho z = 1.82 \times 10^{-2}$ gram cm^{-2} (from total weight of the card divided by its area) and $c = 1.26$ J/(g deg) (heat capacity of cellulose). Then $V \approx 0.186$ cm/s which is of the same order as the observed value of 0.148 cm/s.

If we let $\sigma = \rho zc/2$ be the heat capacity per unit area for a half thickness of the card and set $\epsilon/d = 1.5$, Equation 6 becomes

$$V = 1.5 \frac{\lambda}{\sigma} \frac{(T_f - T_0)}{(T_p - T_0)} \tag{6 a}$$

which is of nearly the same form as that of J. de Ris [5] for the flame spread upwind along a liquid surface, namely

$$V = \sqrt{2} \frac{\lambda}{\sigma} \frac{(T_f - T_v)}{(T_v - T_0)} \tag{6 b}$$

where T_v is the flash point and the other quantities are defined as before. Although both models utilize gas phase heat conduction as the primary heat transfer mechanism, there is a basic difference between them. The present paper considers that most of the heating required to raise the temperature of the surface to the pyrolysis temperature occurs behind the flame front instead of ahead of it.

In the following sections I will describe some experiments which not only justify the concept but determine the values of all the parameters in the first four equations, so that a more careful comparison of the measured and calculated flame spread velocities can be made.

TEMPERATURE MEASUREMENTS IN THE BURNING CARD

The temperature of a point midway between the surfaces of the card was recorded as the flame approached and passed over it. An alumelchromel thermocouple was located in a pocket formed by a scalpel inserted into the card. The relationship between the thermocouple, card and flame is shown in Figure 3. The pocket is located ideally in a neutral plane across which no heat flows so its thermal resistance is unimportant. The card is pressed to form good thermal contact

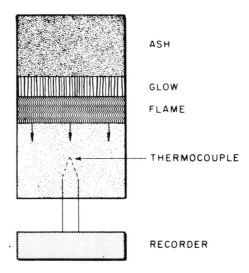

Figure 3. *Location of thermocouple in the white index card.*

between the thermocouple and the card. There was essentially no difference between the results obtained with a 1 mil and a 5 mil thermocouple, so the latter was used because of convenience. In order to evaluate the temperature difference between the center and the surface of the card, the equation for the temperature in a flat plate with a constant heat flux H on one surface and no heat exchange across the other was taken from Carslaw and Jaeger [6]. The second surface corresponds to the mid plane between the two surfaces of the card.

$$T = \frac{H}{\rho c z/2} + \frac{Hz}{2K} \left[\frac{3x^2 - \frac{z^2}{4}}{(3/2)z^2} - \frac{2}{\pi^2} \sum_{n=1}^{\infty} (-1)^n e^{-4\alpha n^2 \pi^2 t/z^2} \cos^2 \frac{n\pi x}{z} \right] \quad (7)$$

Where T is the temperature, H is the irradiance, ρ is the density, c is the heat capacity, z is the thickness of the card, K is the thermal conductivity, x is the distance from the mid plane, q is the thermal diffusivity, and t is the time. On the time scale for downward flame spread the transient term in Equation 7 is negligible.

Letting $x = 0$ and $x = z/2$ we see that the temperature difference between the thermocouple location and the front surface is given by,

$$\Delta T = \frac{Hz}{4K} \quad (8)$$

For H = 2 W/cm², z = 1.2 X 10⁻²cm, and K = 1.2 X 10⁻³ W/(cm deg), ΔT is 5°C.

A typical temperature record is shown in Figure 4. Knowing the velocity of the flame spread and taking the speed of the recorder into account, this temperature history can be converted to a temperature profile at a particular instant. The temperature of the thermocouple when the flame passed over it was noted on the recorder trace and is seen to be about 110°C. This temperature is far too low to contribute a significant amount of pyrolysis products to the atmosphere. Thermogravimetric measurements by Tang and Neil [4] in which cellulose is heated at the low rate of three degree per minute reveal no weight loss below 280°C. Beyond 345° C in Figure 4, there is a pyrolysis plateau where a large part of the heat is going into pyrolysis rather than into the temperature rise of the card. Taking the heat capacity of cellulose to be 1.26 J/(g deg) and the mass per unit area of the card, $\frac{\rho z/2}{2}$, to be 9.1 X 10⁻³ g/cm², and the rate of temperature rise to be 176 deg/s the heat transfer rate to the surface is calculated to be

$$H = \frac{\rho z}{2} c \frac{dT}{dt} = 2.02 \text{ W cm}^{-2} \tag{9}$$

in the linear region. If we assume that heat is being absorbed at the same rate in the pyrolysis region where the rate of temperature rise is only 34 degrees/sec, the rate at which energy is going into pyrolysis is 1.63 W/cm² .

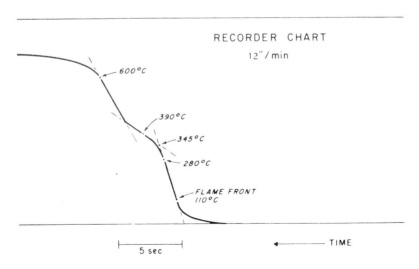

Figure 4. *Temperature history of a point on the card under an advancing flame.*

With a downward flame speed of 0.148 cm/s and a chart speed of 0.5 cm/s (12 inches per minute), the horizontal distances measured on the chart are a factor of 3.4 longer than the vertical distances along the surface of the card. Hence, the pyrolysis zone is seen to be about 3.8 mm long and the flame extension to be about 1.4 mm. This is in good agreement with the visual observations of the flame extension on the burning card. The length of the preheat zone, ϵ, as found by extrapolating the linear portion of the temperature curve back to the time or distance axis is about 2.0 mm. This was verified by adding the flame extension length obtained visually to the thickness of the hot gas zone beyond the flame front found both by thermocouple and shadow graph measurements.

The appearance of the pyrolysis plateau supports the contention that the fuel gases are released behind the flame front rather than ahead of it. To verify that the plateau is indeed due to pyrolysis, the heat of pyrolysis will now be estimated from the measured flame spread velocity and the width of the pyrolysis zone observed in Figure 4. The rate of mass loss per unit area in the pyrolysis zone is given by

$$m = MV/(2WyL) \tag{10}$$

where M is the total mass of the card, V is the velocity of flame spread, L is the length of the card, W is the width of the card and y is the length of the pyrolysis zone. The rate of heat transfer to the surface per unit area effective in producing a temperature rise is given by

$$q = Mc\dot{T}/(2WL) \tag{11}$$

The heat going into pyrolysis per unit area is given by

$$q_p = Mc(\dot{T}_1 - \dot{T}_2)/(2WL) \tag{12}$$

where $\dot{T}_1$ is the rate of temperature rise in the linear region and $\dot{T}_2$ is the rate of temperature rise in the pyrolysis region. The heat of pyrolysis is given by

$$h_p = q_p/m = yc(\dot{T}_i - \dot{T}_2)/V \tag{13}$$

y/V is the time in seconds required from the onset to completion of pyrolysis assuming that the maximum rate applied throughout and would be about 2.5 seconds. With $\dot{T}_1 = 176$ deg/s and $\dot{T}_2 = 34$ deg/s, the heat of pyrolysis is calculated to be 450 J/g which is not far from the value of 368 J/g (88 cal/gram) obtained by Tang and Neil [3] for cellulose in nitrogen using more refined methods.

Cards instrumented in exactly the same way as for the temperature measurements in the flame spread case were inserted into an electric furnace at 600°C which supplied heat directly to the card by radiation in an air environment. The temperature history of a typical card burning in the furnace is shown in Figure 5.

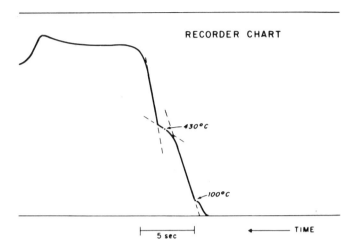

Figure 5. *Temperature history of the card in a furance.*

The similarity of Figures 4 and 5 is striking. The voluminous production of pyrolysis products is observed visually above 400°C leaving no doubt as to the origin of the plateau. The lower plateau at 100°C is due to the driving off of the water.

FLAME SPREAD BURNER

In order to further verify the location of the flame with respect to the pyrolysis zone, to examine the nature of the flame extension in some detail, and to determine the heat transfer rates that could be expected from the flame to the surface, an artificial flame spread surface was constructed in the form of the burner shown in Figure 6. It consists of a water-cooled plenum chamber with replaceable surface plates having 7.5 cm long slots of various widths representing different pyrolysis zones. The burner can be rotated through any desired angle and locked into position. For this work the burner was usually rotated so that the surface plate was oriented in the vertical position. The 3.8 mm pyrolysis zone observed in the card was represented by a 3.2 mm (1/8 inch) slot.

The rate of heat release of the burning pyrolysis gases from each surface of the card is given approximately by

$$q_B = MVQ/2L \qquad (14)$$

Where Q is the heat of combustion of cellulose which is 1.7×10^4 J/g [4]. The factor 1/2 arises because only half of the combustible gases come out from each

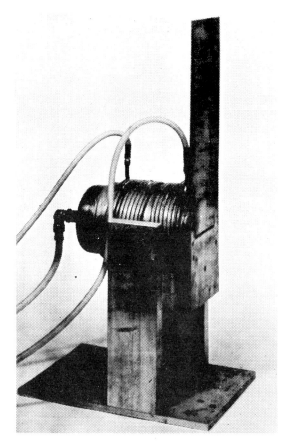

Figure 6. *Flame spread burner.*

surface. The mass of the card is 1.76 g and its length is 12.7 cm. Using the velocity of 0.148 cm/sec, Equation 14 yields 174 watts for the combustion of the pyrolysis gases. The natural gas used in the burner had a heat of combustion of 40 J/cm^3. The gas flow rate was adjusted to 4.4 cm^3/s (0.56 ft^3/hour) in order to match the heat release rate in the flames from the card and the burner. There is no mixing of air with fuel gas prior to its emerging from the slot in the surface plate of the burner.

The similarity of the burning card and the flame spread burner is evident in Figures 7 and 8. In particular, the flame extension and standoff distances are similar. Furthermore, the color of the flame is typically blue in both cases which is characteristic of a premixed flame. This mixing is verified by introducing smoke at the surface beneath the flame. A part of this smoke is drawn in under the flame front.

If the gas flow is increased the upper portion of the flame takes on the yellow

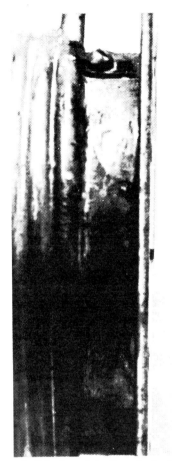

Figure 7. *Side view of the flame in the flame spread burner.*

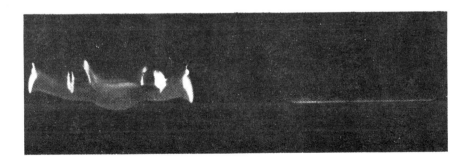

Figure 8. *Comparison of the front views of the flame from the card and the flame from the burner.*

color of a diffusion flame indicating that the air drawn in is insufficient to form a flammable mixture with all of the fuel. The same effect is achieved in the card by merely turning it upside down momentarily to preheat the surface ahead of the flame thereby increasing the fuel supply. The yellow color will persist for a few moments and then disappear.

Below a flow rate of 3.1 cm^3/s (0.40 cu ft per hour), the flame was unstable and would be maintained only briefly. There seems to be a remarkable correlation between this minimum flow and the maximum card thickness which will support downward flame spread. The effect of increasing the thickness is simply to reduce the velocity which should be inversely proportional to thickness according to Equation 4. For two, three, and four card thicknesses, this checks out experimentally except that the flame travels only short distances before extinguishing itself in the case of four thicknesses.

According to Equation 8 the center temperature depression should increase from 5°C to 20°C with four card thicknesses. The rate of pyrolysis of cellulose doubles every 10°C so that the center section is producing pyrolysis gases at only 1/4 the rate of the material at the surface. Integrating over the depth of the specimen, the total pyrolysis rate at the same surface temperature and flame spread velocity is reduced to 56% of its value for a single card, thus the gas flow rate would have to be adjusted for 2.5 cm^3/s which is below the minimum required to maintain a flame.

There is a qualitative correlation between the flame extension and the wind velocity and angle of flame propagation. The extension is increased in the direction of the wind and is decreased on the windward side of the flame. When the opposing air velocity is high enough to eliminate the flame extension for downward propagation the flame extinguishes itself. While other complicating features enter the picture, the length of the extension increases with angle of elevation of the flame as does the flame spread velocity.

The flame spread burner has several advantages for the study of flame spread along surfaces. It provides a fixed stable flame on which many measurements can be made. The pyrolysis rate and width of the pyrolysis zone can be varied which can provide additional insight into the problem. The effect of angle, wind speed, and pressure on the flame shape can be studied apart from their effect on the rate of pyrolysis. The flammability of the fuel gas can be reduced by additives to simulate the effects of flame retardants on the characteristics of the flame.

HEAT TRANSFER TO THE SURFACE

The problem of heat transfer to the surface in the case of flame spread is now reduced to the more general one of determining the heat transfer to the surface beneath the flame. While other heat transfer processes certainly occur to some extent, it appears that in the case of small cellulosic flames gas phase heat conduction is the dominant process and reasonable estimates of the flame spread rate may be obtained by assuming it to be the only one.

In order to estimate the heat transfer to the surface by gas phase heat conduction, the temperature of the gas between the flame and the surface of the flame spread burner was probed with a 1 mil Pt — Pt Rh thermocouple. The horizontal temperature profiles at various distances above and below the bottom edge of the 1/8 inch slot are shown in Figure 9. These thermocouples were not coated to eliminate catalytic effects and were uncorrected for radiation losses. Hence, the temperature profiles are only approximations. The average value of the slopes of these profiles was multiplied by the thermal conductivity of air (4.6×10^{-4} W/(cm deg)) at the average surface temperature (350°C) to obtain a rate of heat transfer of 3.8 W/cm^2. If we assume that this is also the rate of heat transfer from the flame to the card and correct for a radiation loss of 0.5 W/cm^2 at 280°C just before the onset of pyrolysis, we have a net heat transfer to the surface of 3.3 W/cm^2. This is 65% higher than the 2.0 W/cm^2 calculated from the rate of temperature rise in the

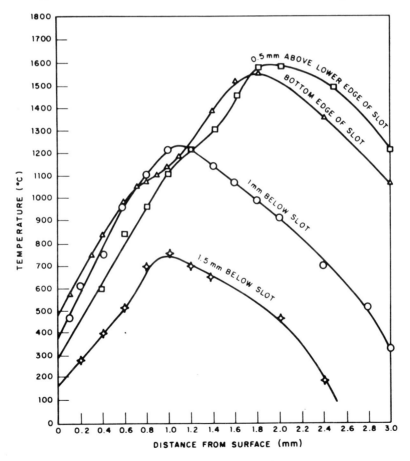

Figure 9. *Horizontal temperature profiles in the flame spread burner.*

card and indicates the plausibility of assuming that the heat transfer to the surface required for flame spread could be supplied by gas phase heat conduction. Because of the difference in flame temperature between the cellulose pyrolysis products and the natural gas and the difference in thermal conductivity of the cellulose surface and the burner surface closer agreement could hardly be expected.

The curves in Figure 9 confirm the presence of the flame at least 1 mm but less than 1.5 mm below the slot (the minimum flame temperature for methane in air is around 1200°C). The visual estimation of the flame extension on the flame spread burner was slightly over 1 mm. The distance below the slot at which paper will ignite is about 1.5 mm which indicates the limit of the preheat zone. The maximum air temperature here according to Figure 9 is about 750°C but is undoubtedly dropping rapidly with distance below the slot. From the width of the luminous band below the pyrolysis zone in Figure 1, the flame extension on the card is estimated to be about 1.5 mm which is in agreement with Figure 4 where the distance between the pyrolysis threshold at 280°C and the passing of the flame front at 110°C is 1.4 mm (based on a chart speed to velocity ratio of 3.4). The ratio of the length of the preheat zone, ϵ, to the flame extension is found to be 1.4 from Figure 4. Multiplying the visual flame extenstion by this ratio, ϵ is calculated to be 2.1 mm. Note that this determination of ϵ is independent of the velocity. The flame extension and preheat zone thus appear to be slightly greater for the card than for the flame spread burner. We are now in a position to estimate the velocity by Equation 4. With $\epsilon = 2.1$ mm, $(\lambda (\frac{\partial T}{\partial x} - \sigma (T^4 - T_0^4)))$ (based on the rate of temperature rise in the card), $T_p - T_0 = 260°C$, $c = 1.26$ J/(g deg) and $\rho z = 1.82 \times 10^{-2}$ g/cm^2, $V = 0.141$ cm/s which is not far from the measured 0.148 cm/s.

The effect of moisture in the cards which were equilibrated to the atmosphere of the laboratory was considered. Drying of the cards results in a 5% weight loss. Taking the latent heat of evaporation of 2260 J/g into account, it was calculated that 113 J/g must be added to the cellulose in order to remove the moisture. In heating a dry card from 20°C to 280°C, 326 J/g are required. We might expect an increase in t_p of 35% and a 26% reduction in velocity according to Equation 1. The velocity in the undried card measures 0.11 cm/s which is in excellent agreement.

The effect of thickness on the velocity of downward flame spread, which was referred to above, was investigated with undried cards stapled together. For 1, 2, 3, and 4 cards the velocities were 0.11 cm/s, 0.052 cm/s, 0.033 cm/s, and 0.023 cm/s inches/min, respectively. The velocity falls off very slightly faster with thickness than is predicted by Equation 4.

CONCLUSIONS

The flame spread mechanism outlined at the beginning of this paper has been justified by the experiments described herein. Pyrolysis has been shown to take place entirely beneath the flame rather than ahead of it. This has been proven by the visual location of the charring surface with respect to the flame, by the temperature of the surface beneath the flame front, by the appearance of a pyrolysis plateau in the temperature history of a point on the card as the flame passes over it, by the appearance of the pyrolysis products from a sample heated to the pyrolysis temperature in a furnace, and by the calculation of the heat of pyrolysis in the burning card which is in rough agreement with that obtained by conventional means. The surface ahead of the pyrolysis zone is heated by the flame directly over it, raising its temperature to the pyrolysis temperature thus causing the flame to move downward. Gas phase heat conduction has been shown to be a plausible mechanism for heating the surface under the flame by showing that the heat transfer calculated from the temperature gradients between the flame and the surface of the flame spread burner are somewhat greater than that calculated from the rate of temperature rise in the card. The maximum thickness for which a specimen will propagate a flame downward has been related to the minimum fuel gas flow which will support a flame. The flame spread burner has emerged as a useful tool in studying flame spread.

By establishing the mechanism for downward flame spread along a thin cellulosic material this work paves the way for a more rigorous treatment of the problem. A satisfactory flame spread theory must be capable of predicting the flame spread velocity completely in terms of the thermal, chemical, and physical properties of the material and the atmosphere rather than partly in terms of such parameters as the preheating length and flame standoff distance which would have to be measured for each application. Hence, the theory should predict these latter parameters as an intermediate step.

Although this paper has been devoted to a very limited facet of flame spread in terms of direction, size, and material there is every reason to believe that the basic mechanism is considerably more general. That is the pyrolysis will generally take place under the flame and heat transfer to the surface will be largely by heat conduction. However, in case of large fires radiation heating ahead of the flame will become an important factor if the emissivity of the flame is sufficiently high.

I wish to acknowledge the help of Mr. Lyman L. Wiltshire for the temperature measurements in the card, and LTJG W. A. O'Hara for the temperature measurements in the gas.

REFERENCES

1. R. Friedman, "A Survey of Knowledge about Idealized Fire Spread over Surfaces," *Fire Research Abstracts and Reviews,* Vol. 10, No. 1, p. 1 (1968).
2. R. M. Fristrom and A. A. Westenberg, "Flame Structure," McGraw Hill, Inc. (1965), p. 284.
3. B. Lewis and G. von Elbe, "Combustion, Flames, and Explosions of Gases," Academic Press, Inc., 1961, p. 281.
4. W. K. Tang and W. K. Neil, "Effect of Flame Retardants on Pyrolysis and Combustion of α-Cellulose," Journal of Polymer Science: Part C, No. 6, p. 65 (1964).
5. J. deRis, "The Spread of a Diffusion Flame over a Thin Combustible Surface," *Fire Research Abstracts and Reviews,* Vol. 10, No. 1, p. 111 (1968).
6. H. S. Carslaw and J. C. Jaeger, "Conduction of Heat in Solids," Oxford University Press (1959), 2nd Edition, p. 112.

W. J. Parker

William J. Parker is a Physicist in the Fire Research Section at the National Bureau of Standards. He received his M.S. degree in Physics at the University of Oregon in 1954. He worked in the Thermal Radiation Branch of the Naval Radiological Defense Laboratory in San Francisco before coming to NBS in 1969. His experience includes U.V., visible, and IR spectroscopy, research on the thermophysical properties of solids, and fire research.

Kogaku Komamiya

The Research Institute of Industrial Safety
Ministry of Labour, Japan
5-35-1 Shiba, Minato-ku, Tokyo, Japan

QUENCHING DISTANCE FOR A COMBUSTIBLE SOLID IN THE OXYGEN-ENRICHED ATMOSPHERE

(Received June 9, 1972)

ABSTRACT: In connection with fire prevention in oxygen-enriched atmosphere, "flame quenching distances" of various combustible solids are measured.

Membranous specimens such as plastic sheets and papers are held between two metal plates having a V- shaped notch, and are ignited at the open end in the combustion chamber in which the pressure is at 1–5 bar. The quenching distance is determined from the width of the notch where the flame ceases to spread.

The results obtained have a good reproducibility and show that the quenching distance can be used as an effective measure for combustibility of solid materials.

In this paper, the details of experimental apparatus and procedure are described, and the correlation between the quenching distance and the "oxygen-index" is discussed.

INTRODUCTION

AS IS WELL known, the combustion of solid materials such as plastic, wood and paper are quenched when they contact a cool body.

This phenomenon is considered to be caused by the heat loss from burning solid. It has fully studied for flame propagation in an explosive gas mixture [1], and the results are utilized in the design of flame arresters But, no or little study has ever been made for the flammable solids[1].

From such standpoint, the quenching distance of membranous solid in oxygen-enriched atmosphere is investigated here experimentally. The results show that the quenching distance becomes an effective measure for combustibility of solids as well as explosive gas mixtures.

EXPERIMENTAL

Apparatus

For supporting the combustible specimen, the brass holder shown in Figure 1 is

---

[1] Recently the author became aware of R. L. Durfee and J. M. Spurlock's report [2] for the plastics burning in oxygen under a reduced-pressure. But their test method is different from that of the author.

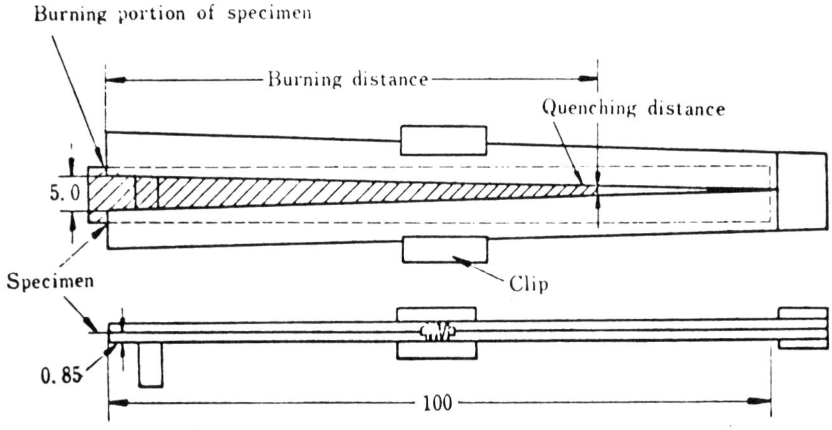

Figure 1. *Holder for measuring quenching distance.*

used. The holder consists of two parts of upper and lower plate with the cut area of "V" shape. The specimen is inserted between these plates, which are then fastened tightly together by means of clips. Thus the test specimen sandwiched between two metal plates has a combustible area of an equilateral triangle whose base is the starting lines of flame spread.

The combustion vessel used for the present experiment is shown in Figure 2. A cover with a glass window is provided for visual observations. A Bourdon type pressure gauge, a valve for supplying an oxidizing gas and an ignition heater were installed at the positions shown in the figure.

Experimental Procedure

A piece of Japanese paper (a sort of paper which is made peculiarly and traditionally in Japan and composed of almost pure cellulose about 10 X 5 mm) is used as ignition aid at the end of a test specimen. The holder prepared with a test specimen is fixed horizontally in the combustion vessel, and after the vessel is closed and purged, the oxidizing gas is introduced through a valve up to a preselected pressure. The following five oxidizing gas mixtures are used: (1) 21%O_2 79%N_2, (2) 42.5%O_2 57.5%N_2, (3) 58.1%O_2 41.9%N_2, (4) 76.3%O_2 23.7%N_2, (5) 100%O_2. Oxygen concentration is measured by gas-interferometer, but the decrease of it in the course of burning is negligible.

The paper is first ignited, the flame then propagates along the test specimen. The flame spread stops at a certain distance depending on the properties of specimen and atmosphere. The length beyond which the flame ceases to propagate denotes the "burning distance," and the minimum width of the burning area at this length is the "quenching distance." The former is measured by a vernier calipers and the latter is calculated from the burning distance.

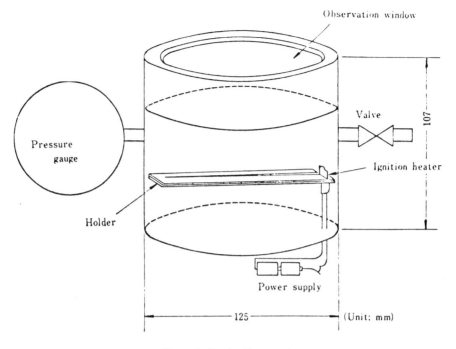

Figure 2. *Combustion vessel.*

Specimens

The characteristics of test specimens used are shown in Table 1. These are mostly commercial ones and the amounts of the additives and the plasticizer are not determined. The sizes of specimens are 25 X 200 mm for the case when air is used as the atmosphere, and 7 X 100 mm for other cases. The specimens are cut from rolled film in the direction perpendicular to the axis of the roll. Also, the test specimens were kept in a silica gel desiccator for over two days before experiment.

RESULTS

Quenching Distance of Various Materials

Quenching distance and burning distance are measured for various materials in an atmosphere of 100% oxygen at 1 bar. Results obtained are summarized in Table 2 (mean value of three trials). As seen in this table, the quenching distance of polyethylene or Japanese paper is very small in comparison with the hydrocarbon polymers containing halogen as polytetrafluoroethylene. Also polychloro-trifluoroethylene was difficult to measure in the oxygen of atmospheric pressure because of a high flame resistance.

It is an interesting fact that the quenching distances for these combustible materials are near those of explosive gases.

Table 1. Characteristics of Specimens

Specimen	Shape	Process	Weight per unit section (g/cm^2)	Thickness (mm)
Japanese paper	Paper		0.00105	0.05
Polyethylene	Film	Extrusion	0.0046	0.05
Nomex	Paper		0.0040	0.055
Polyethyleneterephthalate	Biaxial oriented film	Extrusion	0.0071	0.055
Cellulose triacetate	Film	Casting	0.0065	0.05
Polyvinylchloride	Film	Extrusion	0.0058	0.05
Polyvinylidenefluoride	Biaxial oriented film	Extrusion	0.0114	0.05
Polyvinylidenechloride	Tubular film	Extrusion	0.0065	0.04
Fluorinated ethylene propylene-FEP100	Tubular film	Extrusion	0.07	0.34
Polytetrafluoroethylene	Film	Slicing	0.010	0.05
Polychlorotrifluoroethylene	Film	Extrusion	0.025~0.05	0.15~0.3
Carbon fiber	Paper non-woven		0.013	0.25

Table 2. Burning and Quenching Distances of Various Materials
$(1kg/cm^2, 100\%0_2, Horizontal Spread)$

Specimen	Mean burning distance (mm)	Mean quenching distance (mm)	State of flame
Japanese paper	86.8	0.66	Blue flame
Polyethylene	85.1	0.75	Blue flame
Nomex	85.0	0.75	Change into glow combustion on the way
Polyethyleneterephthalate	81 2	0.94	Bright flame
Cellulose triacetate	79.9	1.01	Bright flame
Polyvinylchloride	77 2	1 14	Bright flame accompanied by soot
Polyvinylidenefluoride	74.4	1 28	Bright flame
Polyvinylidenechloride	57.3	2.14	Red and short flame accompanied by white smoke
Carbon Fiber	17.2	4.14	Glow combustion
Fluorinated ethylene propylene-FEP100	13.0	4.35	Bright carbon particles in blue flame
Polytetrafluoroethylene	6.5	4.68	Bright carbon particles in blue flame
Polychlorotrifluoroethylene	(26.7)*	(3.67)*	A candle like flame

$(*2kg/cm^2)$

Effect of the Holder Plate Thickness

In order to see the effect of the plate thickness, holders with four different thicknesses were tested. Results obtained from these measurements for polyethylene and Japanese paper are shown in Table 3. According to these results it is found that the plate thickness has considerable effect. In this study, a brass holder with a plate thickness of 0.85 mm was used.

Table 3. Effect of Plate Thickness on Burning Distance
(1kg/cm², Horizontal Spread, Unit mm)

Specimen	Oxygen (Vol %)	Plate thickness (mm)				
		0.85	1.0	3.0	9.0	16.0
Polyethylene (mean)	100	85.0	86.0	73.6	63.9	62.8
		85.2	85.5	72.2	62.5	63.4
		85.0	86.0	71.8	65.0	64.9
		(85.1)	(85.8)	(72.5)	(63.8)	(63.7)
Japanese paper (mean)	100	87.0	86.7	77.6	76.0	
		86.8	86.6	77.2	77.3	
		86.5	87.0	78.4	76.8	
		(86.8)	(86.8)	(77.7)	(76.7)	
Japanese paper (mean)	air	31.8	27.6	16.7	14.6	
		32.9	26.2	16.2	14.4	
		32.0	27.6	17.3	14.8	
		(32.2)	(27.1)	(16.7)	(14.6)	

Effect of the Specimen Thickness

The effects of specimen thickness on the quenching distance are examined by using multilayered sheets. The fuels tested were Japanese paper and polyethylene. The results shown in Table 4 indicate that the quenching distance is not greatly influenced by the specimen thickness. The burning time from ignition to quenching, however, increases with the increase in number of sheets.

Table 4. Effect of Specimen Thickness on Burning Distance
(1kg/cm², 100%O_2, Horizontal Spread, Unit mm)

Specimen	Number of piled sheets			
	1	2	4	6
Polyethylene	85.1	84.5	81.7	
Japanese paper	86.8	86.4	85.7	85.8

Effect of Orientation

The effect of orientation was studied by considering the following four cases: (1) upward vertical, (2) downward vertical, (3) longitudinal-horizontal and (4) horizontal directions (see Figure 3). The test fuels are once again Japanese paper and polyethylene and the atmosphere was an oxygen-nitrogen mixture with 40.7%

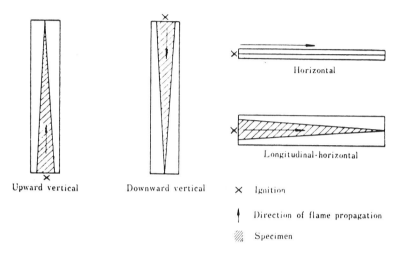

Figure 3. *Orientation of flame propagation (side-views).*

oxygen under 1 bar. The results obtained are shown in Table 5. For Japanese paper, the burning distance decreases in the order of upward vertical, longitudinal horizontal, downward vertical, and horizontal direction. This behavior is similar to the flame propagation in an explosive gas. For polyethylene, on the other hand, the burning distance decreases in the order of downward vertical, longitudinal horizontal, upward vertical, and horizontal directions. This discrepant behavior is noted to be mostly due to the dripping melt.

Table 5. *Relationship Between Orientation and Burning Distance (1kg/cm² , Unit mm)*

Specimen	Oxygen (Vol %)	Upward Vertical	Longitudinal Horizontal	Downward Vertical	Horizontal
Polyethylene	40.7	68.3	68.9	69.9	66.2
Japanese paper	air	39.2	30.6	28.7	25.6

Effects of the Oxygen Concentration and Pressure

The burning distance for different oxygen concentration and pressures is measured in the horizontal direction for polyethylene, polyvinylchloride, and polytetrafluoroethylene. The results are shown in Figures 4 and 5. In these tests, the

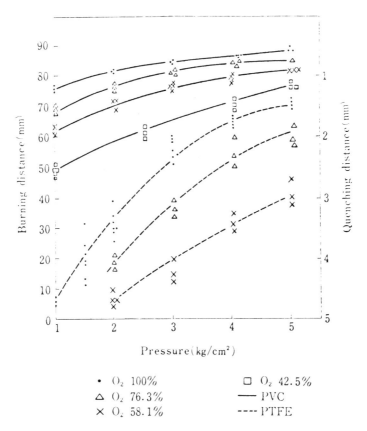

Figure 4. *Effect of oxygen concentration and pressure on quenching distance of polyethylene (horizontal spread).*

reproducibility was inferior for polytetrafluoroethylene due to the fact that the test specimen was prepared by slicing, so its surface was quite irregular microscopically. The quenching distance decreases with the pressure and the oxygen concentration. Usually the effect of the latter is far larger than that of the former. For example, the quenching distance corresponding to air at a pressure of 5 bar is about 1.87 mm. On the other hand, corresponding to pure oxygen at a total pressure of 1 bar, it is about 0.75 mm. If combustion is controlled by the partial pressure of oxygen, these two quenching distance measurements should be equal to one another. The

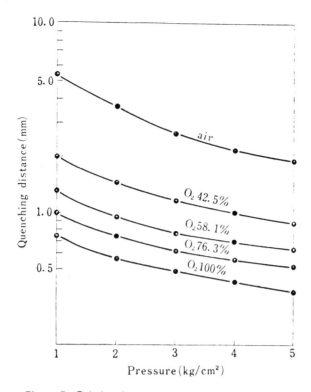

Figure 5. *Relation between oxygen concentration and/or pressure and burning distance of polyvinylchloride and poly-tetrafluoroethylene (horizontal spread).*

great difference between the two values suggests that the combustion of solid materials does not depend solely on the oxygen partial pressure.

Flame Separation Phenomenon in Polyvinylchloride

In the experiments on polyvinylchloride, the flame is observed to be separated into two stages in the range of oxygen concentration of 40–50%. The first flame is associated with the first step of the PVC pyrolysis whereas the second flame is connected with a burning of the residue. The second flame is quenched earlier than the first one. The detailed mechanism of this interesting phenomenon is not yet understood. A sketch obtained from the experiment is given in Figure 6.

COMPARISON WITH OXYGEN-INDEX METHOD

As a means for measuring the combustibility of solid materials, the limiting oxygen-index method developed by Fenimore and Martin [3] is very useful and many measured LOI values have been previously published [4, 5, 6].

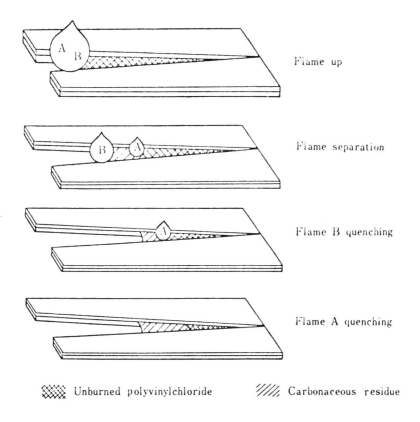

Flame up

Flame separation

Flame B quenching

Flame A quenching

▨ Unburned polyvinylchloride   ▨ Carbonaceous residue

Figure 6. *Flame separation of polyvinylchloride (0_2 42.5%, $1kg/cm^2$, horizontal spread).*

This method based on the critical oxygen concentration of the atmosphere at which the specimen ignited by a pilot flame can be kept to burn, has a disadvantage that it is impossible to obtain the index for highly flame resistant materials such as polychlorotrifluoroethylene because the oxygen-index becomes greater than 100.

On the other hand, the present method based on the quenching distance can be applied to any material by the control of ambient pressure, for example the quenching distance of above-mentioned flame resistant polymer is easily determined as 3.67 mm under an atmospheric pressure of 2 bar. Moreover, as shown in Figure 7, the results obtained by this experimental procedure correlate fully well with the oxygen-index.

In Figure 7, the oxygen-indices reported by Isaacs [4] are plotted with the present quenching distances on a semilogarithmic diagram. It is clear from this figure that the relationship between the two measures of flammability follows law.

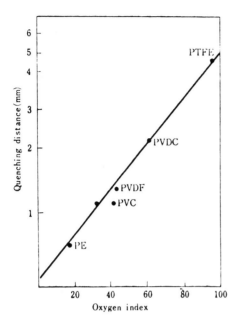

Figure 7. *A relationship between quenching distance and oxygen index (all these quenching distances are for 100% oxygen 1.0 kg/cm²).*

SUMMARY

From the above experimental results, we can conclude that the quenching distance is a useful measure to compare the combustibility of solid materials. The new method has the advantage of simplicity and good reproducibility while correlating well with Fenimore and Martin's oxygen-index method.

The author is thankful to Dr. K. Akita, University of Tokyo, for helpful discussions.

REFERENCES

1. B. Lewis, G. Von Elbe, "Combustion, Flames and Explosions of Gases," Academic Press (1961) pp. 228, 328.
2. R. L. Durfee, J. M. Spurlock, "Quenching and Extinguishment of Burning Solids in Oxygen Enriched Atmospheres," Contract No. NAS9–8470, Atlantic Research Corporation (1969).
3. C. P. Fenimore, F. J. Martin, "Flammability of Polymers," Combustion and Flame, *10*, 135, (1966).
4. J. L. Isaacs, "The Oxygen Index Flammability Test," J. Fire & Flammability, *1*, 36, (1970).
5. K. Komamiya, "Flammability of Fabrics," Kasai (Journal of Fire Prevention Society of Japan), *12*, 75, (1962) (in Japanese).
6. K. Komamiya, "Flammability Test of Plastics Films," Anzen Kogaku (Journal of Japan Society for Safety Engineering), *2*, 270, (1963) (in Japanese).

J. M. FUNT AND J. H. MAGILL

Department of Metallurgical and Materials Engineering
University of Pittsburgh
Pittsburgh, Pennsylvania 15213

APPLICATION OF A FLAME-SPREAD MODEL
TO THE OXYGEN INDEX TEST

(Received January 18, 1973)

ABSTRACT: Using the model developed by McAlevy and co-workers, the burning velocity in vertically-downward burning can be predicted by the equation

$$V = 2 \frac{\left[k_g \triangle H\, P^a\, Y_{ox}^{1+b} \right] 2}{k_s\, P_s C_s^2\, C_g\, \ell\, (T_s - T_o)^2}$$

This equation satisfactorily predicted the burn rate of polystyrene films using an oxygen-index of 20–50%, g as velocity of 6–17 cm/min, film thickness of 5–20 mils and using either nitrogen or helium as the inert diluent.

INTRODUCTION

IN THE PROPER engineering design of materials for construction and other uses, consideration must be given to the flame resistance of the materials as well as physical properties. The most widely used general test for this purpose is the Limiting Oxygen Index Test [1]. Specific ASTM tests have been designed for application in specific industries as well [2]. The new Federal regulations being promulgated for fire safety [3] are similar in philosophy to the ASTM tests in that they attempt to simulate fire behavior under in-use conditions. One of the limitations to the study of polymer flammability by these types of tests is that it is not clear exactly what processes the test measures.

Combustion is a complex physical and chemical process [4]. Not only does it depend on chemical and physicochemical effects such as reactive species and bond strengths, but it also depends on purely aerodynamic effects such as rates of heat and rates of mass convection [5]. In the flammability tests mentioned above, it is difficult to separate these processes in order to determine the effect of material properties independently of the effect of aerodynamic variables. In the modification of the oxygen index test described below, a method for the separation of these effects is described.

THE FLAME SPREAD MODEL

In this model, originally derived by McAlevy and co-workers, [6] a heat balance is made between the heat released in the gas-phase combustion reaction and the heat required to raise the surface temperature of the burning polymer to the pyrolysis temperature.

The physical picture of the model is given in Figure 1. As the flame traverses the

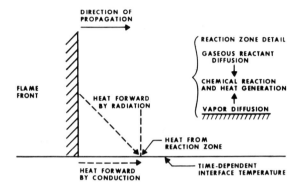

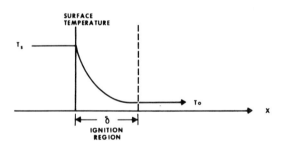

Figure 1. *Physical basis of the flame spread model (after McAlevy and Magill (6a)).*

polymer surface, the polymer is heated ahead of the flame. This heat transfer raises the surface temperature significantly over a short distance only, the ignition region δ. As the flame passes a point in its path, the temperature here reaches a fixed value, T_s, which is the temperature required to pyrolyze the polymer in sufficient quantities to sustain the flame. The surface temperature in the flame zone then remains constant until all of the fuel is consumed.

The gas-phase heat conservation equation for a quiescent atmosphere is

$$\alpha \frac{\partial^2 T_g}{\partial y^2} = -\frac{\triangle H}{\rho_g C_{p,g}} C_f C_{ox} A \exp(-E/RT)$$

where
y	$=$	coordinate perpendicular to the surface
α	$=$	gas thermal diffusivity $= k_g/\rho_g C_{p,g}$
H	$=$	heat of combustion
ρ_g	$=$	gas density
$C_{p,g}$	$=$	heat capacity of the gas
k_g	$=$	thermal conductivity
C_f, C_{ox}	$=$	concentration of fuel and oxidant
A, E	$=$	Arrhenius rate constants
T	$=$	temperature

The gas-phase mass conservation equation for a quiescent atmosphere is

$$D \frac{\partial^2 C_f}{\partial y^2} = C_{ox} C_f A \exp(-E/RT)$$

where D = diffusivity.

As a first approximation, the effects of bulk gas-phase convection are neglected to simplify the mathematics. The convection effects will be included as an empirical correction to the solution for diffusion only.

Solution of the coupled gas-phase equations gives

$$Q_s = k_g Y_{ox} \triangle H \, F(P_2 Y_{ox}) C_{p,g}^{-1}$$

where
Q_s	$=$	heat flux to the surface
Y_{ox}	$=$	oxygen index $= \dfrac{C_{ox}}{C_{ox} + C_{inert}}$
F	$=$	$P^a Y_{ox}^b$, a, b constants

The solid phase energy conservation equation is

$$\frac{\partial T'}{\partial t} = \frac{k_s}{\rho_s, C_{p,s}} \frac{\partial^2 T'}{\partial y^2}$$

where
T'	$=$	$T_{(y,t)} - T_o$
T_o	$=$	initial temperature
$k_s, \rho_s, C_{p,s}$	$=$	thermal conductivity, density and heat capacity of solid

This equation has two solutions [6, 7]. If the thermal penetration is comparable to the fuel bed thickness, then

$$Q_s = \rho_s C_{p,s} V \, \mathfrak{t} \, (T_s - T_o)$$

95

where V =   flame spread velocity

                    T_s =   surface temperature at the flame

                    $\uparrow$ =   fuel bed thickness

If the fuel bed thickness is greater than the thermal penetration thickness, then

$$Q_s = 0.89 \, (k_s \, \rho_s \, C_s \, V)^{1/2} \, (T_s - T_o)$$

Equating the heat flux from the gas-phase to the solid phase and solving for the flame spread velocity [6]

$$V = \frac{2 \, k_g \, \triangle H \, Y_{ox} F(P, Y_{ox})}{\rho_s \, C_s \, C_g \, \uparrow \, (T_s - T_o)} \qquad \text{thin beds}$$

$$V = \frac{2 \left[k_g \, \triangle H \, Y_{ox} \, F \, (P, \, Y_{ox}) \right]^2}{k_s \rho_s C_s^2 \, C_g \, \uparrow (T_s - T_o)^2} \qquad \text{thick beds}$$

Although these equations were derived for flame spread over the surface of a fuel bed, the boundary condition

$$\frac{dT'}{d\chi} = 0 \text{ at } x = 0$$

is met for a burning film if the film midplane is the $x = 0$ plane.

The key assumptions in this derivation are equating the two heat fluxes and neglecting boundary layer effects. Other derivations have been made using these same assumptions and, although the mathematics appear different, the solutions are essentially equivalent [8, 9].

These equations were derived assuming no bulk gas phase convection. If the gas phase is flowing so that bulk convection effects become important, the predicted burn rate is [6]

$$V = V'U_g^{1/3}$$

where V' =   burn rate for diffusion only

                    U_g =   bulk gas velocity

This is an empirical correction for the neglect of mass transport of the oxidant by bulk convection.

The experimental results reported here are a test of this model in the case of candle-like burning of polystyrene films. If the derivation is applicable, then the material flammability properties can be separated from the aerodynamic effects.

EXPERIMENTAL PROCEDURE

The test materials were obtained from Koppers Corporation, and consisted of polystyrene sheets with constant thickness of 5, 10 and 20 mils respectively.

Oxygen was used as the oxidant gas and helium and/or nitrogen were employed as the inert gas.

The measurements were made on a TRI Flammability Analyzer, available from Custom Scientific Corporation. This apparatus uses the polymer film strapped to a wheel and rotated by a variable speed motor (Figure 2). The film was ignited by a methane flame from a bunsen burner. The apparatus, described by Miller, [10] enables one to measure the burn rate using any desired direction of burn. In our

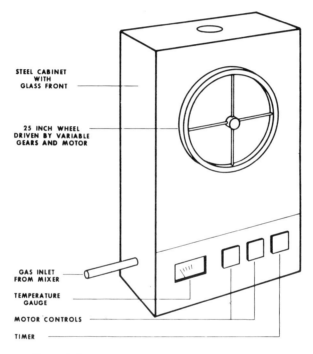

STEEL CABINET
WITH
GLASS FRONT

25 INCH WHEEL
DRIVEN BY VARIABLE
GEARS AND MOTOR

GAS INLET
FROM MIXER

TEMPERATURE
GAUGE

MOTOR CONTROLS

TIMER

Figure 2. *Schematic view of tri-flammability apparatus.*

experiments, vertically downward burning was used because the model does not predict the effect of surface preheating by convected combustion gases.

The controlled experimental parameters were film thickness, inert species, oxygen concentration and gas stream velocity. The ranges of these variables are given in Table 1. The effect of changing the inert gas species is to alter the gas phase properties without altering the reaction mechanism.

RESULTS

The experimental results are presented in Table 1. For each run, the burn velocity was measured as a function of film thickness, gas phase composition and gas velocity.

Table 1. Evaluation of a Flame Spread Model

Material: Polystyrene   P = 14.7 psia

T_o = 25 ± 2° C

Film Thickness (mils)	Gas Velocity (cm/min)	Oxygen Index (% O_2)	Inert Species	Burn Rate (cm/min)
5	6.1	20	N_2	9.5
5	6.1	35	N_2	21
5	6.1	50	N_2	37
5	9.8	20	N_2	12
5	9.8	35	N_2	27
5	9.8	50	N_2	47
5	13.5	20	N_2	14
5	13.5	35	N_2	29
5	13.5	50	N_2	67
10	6.1	20	N_2	7
10	6.1	35	N_2	14
10	6.1	50	N_2	28
10	9.8	35	N_2	15
10	9.8	50	N_2	21
10	13.5	20	N_2	15
10	13.5	35	N_2	14
10	13.5	50	N_2	27
20	6.1	20	N_2	8
20	6.1	50	N_2	14
20	9.8	20	N_2	8
20	9.8	35	N_2	11
20	9.8	50	N_2	15
20	13.5	20	N_2	13
20	13.5	50	N_2	15
5	9.8	20	He	17
5	9.8	35	He	28
5	9.8	50	He	51
5	13.5	20	He	23
5	13.5	35	He	34
5	13.5	50	He	46
5	17.2	20	He	21
5	17.2	35	He	36
10	9.8	20	He	11
10	9.8	35	He	17
10	13.5	20	He	16
10	13.5	35	He	21
10	13.5	50	He	36
10	17.2	20	He	13
10	17.2	35	He	20
10	17.2	50	He	32

Several trends in the data are discernible. For constant film thickness, inert species and gas velocity, the burn rate increases with increased oxygen index. For constant inert species, gas velocity and oxygen index, the burn rate then decreases with increased film thickness. For constant inert species, film thickness and oxygen index, the burn rate increases with increased gas velocity. Finally, the burn rate increases when helium is substituted for nitrogen with all other variables constant.

All of the independent variables can be combined in accordance with the model predicted for thick films, using the values of $a = 0.2$ and $b = 0.14$, as determined by McAlevy from surface burning data [6]. For the case of $O_2 - N_2$, a value of $2 \triangle H^2 / (T_s - T_o)^2 = 5.0 \times 10^3$ was used. A comparison of the experimental and calculated values of the burn rate is shown in Figure 3. However, one exception

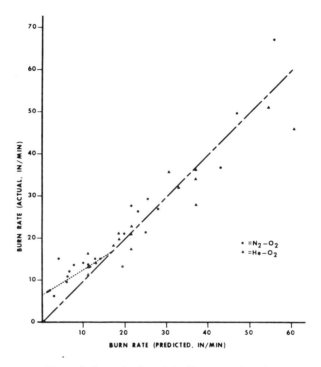

Figure 3. *An evaluation of the flame spread model.*

must be noted. For low oxygen index values in helium, where mass transport by diffusion is rapid compared to that in nitrogen, the convection correction term drops out. Under these conditions, the experimental burn rate is consistently higher than the predicted burn rate for low values of the burn rate. All of these experimental points correspond to an oxygen index of 0.20 which is close to the limiting oxygen index of 0.19. In this region, the boundary layer becomes fuel rich and the

combustion reaction becomes pseudo-first order, independent of fuel concentration
[11]. Then the value of (a) becomes 0 for Y_{ox} near the limiting oxygen index, and
the fit to experimental results is improved (Figure 4).

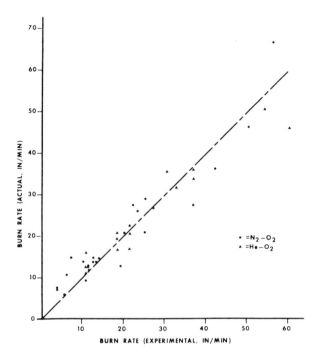

Figure 4. *An evaluation of the modified flame spread model.*

DISCUSSION

The display in Figure 4 shows a reasonable correlation between the predicted
burn rate and the experimental results. Because polystyrene flows readily at the
surface temperatures involved, it was impossible to obtain a good measurement of
the surface temperature T_s using a thermocouple. However, TGA analysis indicates
that T_s should be near 350–400°C. With a value of $T_s = 350$°C, H can be calculated
as 1.6×10^6 cal/mole styrene monomers [12]. This shows that the empirical
parameter $\triangle H/ (T_s - T_o)$ has an acceptable value. At the present time, it is
impossible to determine if the change in this parameter with inert species is caused
by experimental error or by actual changes in $\triangle H$ or T_s. Because the only change in
the system is the thermal constants of the gaseous mixture due to a change of
inerts, $\triangle H/ (T_s - T_o)$ should remain constant. Therefore, the observed apparent
variation is probably caused by experimental error or arises because of the approximate form of the model.

That the model is only approximate is shown by the necessity of using two values of (a) and two values of the exponent of U_g. Although these changes can be rationalized qualitatively from the physical arguments given above, an exact model should predict these changes.

To obtain a more realistic model of the burning process, it is necessary to solve the boundary layer equations for coupled heat and mass transfer through a turbulent boundary layer with transverse diffusion and chemical reaction. Some progress has been made in obtaining solutions to this problem, [13] but no analytical solution has been obtained yet.

The advantage of our model is that the important controllable parameters and the material properties are considered explicitly. Even though the model is semi-empirical, it does indicate that the effect of material properties on burn rates can be separated from aerodynamic effects.

Although all the measurements necessary to quantitatively verify the model were not made, the results of Miller, [10] Nakakuki [14] and Welker [15] agree qualitatively with the predictions of the model.

Miller [10] examined the burning rate of a variety of textile materials as a function of fabric weight and oxygen index. The burning rate varied approximately as the first order with respect to oxygen index and approximately as the inverse first order with respect to the fabric weight, which is the behavior expected for "thin" samples.

Nakakuki [14] examined the effect of oxygen index and pressure on the flame spread rate. He found that the burning rate depended on these variables as

$$V = A \, Y_{ox}{}^m \, P^n$$

The values of m and n for several materials are given in Table 2. Not only is the power law dependence the same as predicted by this model, but the values of m and n are those expected for a thick fuel bed.

Table 2. Power Law Parameters for Burn Velocities [14]

$$V = A \, Y_{ox}{}^m P^n$$

Material	Mode of Burn	A	m	n	Pressure range (atm.)
Cypress	Horizontal	2.63	2.45	0.71	1–3
Rayon Cloth	45° Down	19.2	2.80	0.73	1–2
Vinyl Cord	Horizontal	1.74	1.99	0.52	1–3
Filter Paper	45° Down	2.19	1.66	0.75	1–2
	Horizontal	2.54	1.59	0.60	

Welker [15] examined the important parameters for the ignition of polymers by radiant energy. By postulating that the sample would ignite when the surface temperature had reached a given value, dependent on the type of material, he was able to construct a model which predicted the time to ignition based on material properties. This agrees with the physical basis of our model which assumes that the flame front will pass a point when the surface temperature has reached some definite level.

Several deficiencies are evident in the results presented here, but work is now planned which will correct these. First, the ambient temperature, T_0, had only one value. The apparatus is now being modified to allow the measurement of burn rates at elevated temperatures.

The parameters $\triangle H$ and T_s should be measured independently and then used in the model to predict the burn rate. A modified DTA apparatus which will allow both of these variables to be measured using small samples is being constructed. If this type of test can provide values of H and T_s which correctly predict the burning behavior in the oxygen index test, then a simple thermal analysis may be able to replace a wide variety of small-scale flame tests which cannot be readily correlated at the present time. More importantly, it appears that H and T_s will be significant parameters in predicting flame hazard using models of *in-use situations* such as are now being developed by workers at Factory Mutual Corporation [16].

Once our model has been verified for polystyrene films, various polymers and flame retardants will be examined. A study of the change of H and T_s with fuel materials should give some insight into the mechanism of flame retardance and should suggest means of reducing the intrinsic flammability of polymers. Work to this end is now in progress.

ACKNOWLEDGMENTS

Financial support for this project has been supplied by the Pennsylvania Science and Engineering Foundation. The polymer samples have been provided by Mr. R. Kratz of Sinclair-Koppers Corporation, Pittsburgh.

REFERENCES

1. J. L. Isaacs, J. Fire and Flammability, *1*, 36 (1970).
2. C. J. Hilado, Polymer Conference Series on Polymer Flammability, University of Detroit, 1970.
3. Federal Register, November 12, 1971.
4. R. Fristrom and A. A. Westenberg, *Flame Structure* (New York: McGraw-Hill Book Co., 1965).
5. F. A. Williams, *Combustion Theory* (Reading, Mass.: Addison-Wesley Publishing Co., 1965).
6. F. A. Lasterina, R. S. Magee, R. F. McAlevy, Thirteenth Symposium (International) on Combustion, 935 (1971).
6a. R. F. McAlevy, R. S. Magee, Twelfth Symposium (International) on Combustion, 215 (1969).
7. H. D. Carslaw, J. C. Jeager, *Conduction in Solids*, 2nd Ed. (Clarendon Press, 1959).

8. J. N. DeRis, Twelfth Symposium (International) on Combustion, 241 (1969).
9. C. Sanchez Tarifa, P. Perez del Notario, M. Torralbo, Twelfth Symposium (International) on Combustion, 229 (1969).
10. B. Miller, Polymer Conference Series on Polymer Flammability, University of Detroit, 1970.
11. L. Green, in *Heterogeneous Combustion*, H. G. Wolfhard, I. Glassman and L. Green, Eds., p. 451 (New York: Academic Press, 1964).
12. J. M. Smith and H. C. Van Ness, Introduction to Chemical Engineering Thermodynamics, 2nd Ed., p. 138 (New York: McGraw-Hill Book Co., 1959).
13. T. Kashiwagi and M. Summerfield, to be published, Fourteenth Symposium (International) on Combustion, 1972.
14. A. Nakakuki, J. Fire and Flammability, *3*, 146 (1972).
15. J. R. Welker, Polymer Conference Series on Polymer Flammability, University of Detroit, 1970.
16. J. DeRis, Combustion Science and Technology, *2*, 239 (1970).

John M. Funt

John M. Funt received his B.S. and M.Eng. degrees in chemical engineering from Cornell University and his M.S. and Ph.D. degrees from the University of Massachusetts in 1972. He is now a post-doctoral research associate in the Metallurgical and Materials Engineering Department at the University of Pittsburgh.

Joseph H. Magill

Joseph H. Magill received his B.Sc. and Ph.D. degrees from Queens University, Belfast, N. Ireland in 1956. Currently he is an associate professor in the Metallurgical and Materials Engineering Department at the University of Pittsburgh.

A Four-Foot Tunnel Test Apparatus for Measuring Surface Flame Spread

Carlos J. Hilado and Paul E. Burgess, Jr.*

Research and Development Department
Chemicals and Plastics
Union Carbide Corporation
South Charleston, West Virginia 25303

(Received February 11, 1972)

ABSTRACT

A four-foot-long tunnel test apparatus offers substantial reductions in cost of sample preparation and testing, when used as a screening tool for rigid foam samples intended for the ASTM E 84 25-foot tunnel. The reference materials used, asbestos-cement board and Kode 25 rigid foam, exhibit better reproducibility than the red oak prescribed for the ASTM E 84 test, and should be used in calibrating each duplicate tunnel.

The response of Kode 25 to various levels of applied heat flux suggests that flame spread along the surface of a self-extinguishing combustible material may be a linear function of the heat flux applied.

INTRODUCTION

The 25-foot tunnel test developed at Underwriters' Laboratories by Mr. A. J. Steiner [1] has become a widely accepted test for evaluating the surface flame-spread hazard of building and interior finish materials. This test, known as ASTM E 84 [2], UL 723 [3], and NFPA 255 [4], rates materials on a scale on which asbestos-cement board is zero and select-grade red oak flooring is 100. Some arbitrary levels of ratings between these two reference materials are important in that they represent acceptance requirements for certain markets, and hence requirements for penetration of these markets by new or improved materials. A flame-spread rating of 25, for example, gives a Class A or Class 1 rating according to many building codes, and in some cases qualifies the material as "noncombustible." A flame-spread rating of 75 is a requirement for interior finishes in certain types of occupancies such as hospitals.

The 25-foot tunnel test requires a specimen 25 feet long and 20 inches wide, mounted face down so as to form the roof of a 25-foot-long tunnel 17.5 inches wide and 12 inches high. Even on a development basis without certification, the 25-foot tunnel test is much more expensive to run than a small-scale laboratory test, and the specimen required for this test is beyond the scale of the small quantities in which

---

*Mr. Burgess is now with Panacon Corporation, 316 S. Wayne Ave., Cincinnati, Ohio.

most experimental materials are prepared. A need exists to develop the ability to predict the performance of materials in the 25-foot tunnel on the basis of their performance in laboratory tests requiring only small amounts of material. Several tests have been developed and used with limited success, but their predictive abilities appear to be valid only for certain classes of materials and within specific ranges of performance. These tests include the Forest Products Laboratory 8-foot tunnel [5], also known as ASTM E 286 [6], the National Bureau of Standards radiant panel [7], also known as ASTM E 162 [8], the Monsanto 2-foot tunnel [9], the Pittsburgh-Corning 30-inch tunnel [10], and the Butler chimney test [11].

All these smaller-scale flame-spread tests differ significantly from the 25-foot tunnel in one important aspect of geometry: none of them provide for the identical situation of flame spread along the underside of a horizontal surface under conditions of forced convection parallel to the surface. The importance of the angle of inclination of the surface has been discussed [12], and some effects of surface angle have been reported [13]. The smaller-scale tests listed above which have tunnel-type configurations have specimen surfaces inclined from 6 to 30 degrees from the horizontal.

One horizontal test which provides the same geometric position as the 25-foot tunnel is a small tunnel developed by Upjohn for which an empirical relationship was developed based on a large number of samples tested in both the 25-foot and small tunnels. Information on this apparatus, however, is restricted.

A 4-foot laboratory tunnel was built in an effort to develop the ability to predict the performance of materials in the 25-foot tunnel. This apparatus has not been sufficiently developed to serve as a standard test method but is presented as an evaluation tool because of its substantial reductions in costs of screening materials.

CONSTRUCTION AND TRIALS

The specimen surface in the laboratory tunnel is horizontal, so that the Union Carbide tunnel provides the same geometric position for the specimen surface as the 25-foot tunnel. Tunnel dimensions were arbitrarily selected, based on experience with other flammability tests. A length of four feet was selected because this represented a substantial reduction in sample size from the 25-foot tunnel and the 8-foot FPL tunnel.

An exposed specimen width of 6 inches was selected in a compromise between material limitations on experimental samples and the need to reduce edge effects. A tunnel depth of 6 inches was selected, with the result that the length was nominally 1/6 the length of the 25-foot tunnel, the width was 1/3, and the depth was 1/2.

To reduce burner variables, a single-head burner was selected instead of the two-headed burner in the 25-foot tunnel, and the burner was positioned in the lower half of the cross section as in the 25-foot tunnel. Positioning the burner in the upper half of the cross section showed no consistent difference in maximum flame length and hence offered no improvement in the form of a greater range for flame spread measurements.

As in the 25-foot tunnel, air movement was induced by an exhaust blower installed at the vent end. The distance that the flame traveled was viewed through the tunnel bottom which was made of wire glass.

The tunnel is shown in Figures 1, 2, and 3. Figure 1 shows the tunnel with the asbestos-cement board reference material in place. Chromel-alumel thermocouples spaced along the length of the tunnel are used to measure temperatures as a function of distance and time. Figure 2 shows the tunnel with a sample in place, and Figure 3 is an end view showing the burner in place. Variations in dimensions during actual construction resulted in an actual specimen measuring 47.5 inches long and 7.5 inches wide, with an actual exposed area of 46 by 6 inches, and an actual depth of 6.75 inches.

The following approach was used to optimize operating conditions: First, various levels of air supply rate and fuel supply rate were used to determine the effects of scaling down, and an operating range was selected which would provide at least 24 inches of length for flame spread measurements. Second, red oak was used as a reference material to determine the flame spread behavior corresponding to a rating of 100. Third, Upjohn Kode 25 rigid foam was used as a reference material to determine the flame spread behavior corresponding to a rating of 25.

Air was supplied in the 25-foot tunnel at a rate which gave a velocity of 240 feet per minute through the 12 by 17.5 inch cross section. For the 6.375 by 6 inch cross section of the laboratory tunnel, three levels of air velocity were tried: 38.4 feet per minute, which gave the same residence time (6.26 seconds); 240 feet per minute, which gave the same velocity; and 553 feet per minute, which gave the same degree of turbulence (Reynolds number of 33,400).

The initial setting for fuel supply in the 25-foot tunnel involved approximately 5000 Btu per minute. For the laboratory tunnel, three levels of heat supply were tried assuming 2450 Btu/std. cu. ft. for the propane used: 274 Btu per minute, which gave the same heat flux per unit area of exposed specimen surface (137.1 Btu per minute per square foot); 911 Btu per minute, which gave the same heat flux per unit area of tunnel cross section (3429 Btu per minute per square foot); and 1714 Btu per minute, which gave the same heat flux per unit width of specimen (3429 Btu per minute per foot).

Various combinations of air supply rate and fuel supply rate, beginning with the levels previously discussed, were tried. The only combinations which gave flame lengths less than 24 inches seemed to be an air velocity of 157.5 ft/min and a heat supply rate of 274 to 376 Btu per minute. In these trials no air was premixed with the propane in the burner flame.

Trials with red oak specimens showed that a heat supply rate of 376 Btu per minute was not sufficient to produce flaming along the red oak for the full 48 inches, but produced adequate flame spread if air was premixed with the propane in the burner flame to the extent of about 56 percent of stoichiometric.

At the conditions thus arrived at, maximum flame length averaged 17.9 inches (standard deviation 0.7 inch) with asbestos-cement board and 39.5 inches (standard

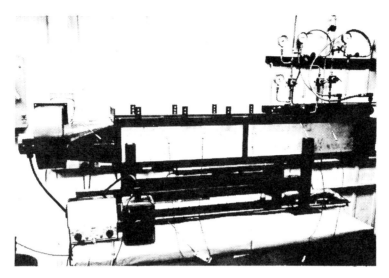

Figure 1. *Four-foot tunnel with asbestos-cement board in place.*

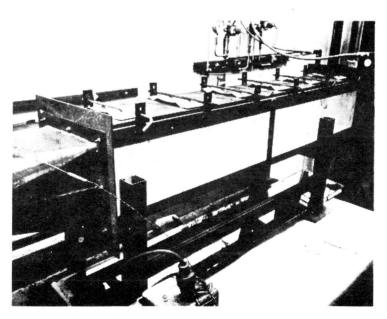

Figure 2. *Four-foot tunnel with test specimen in place.*

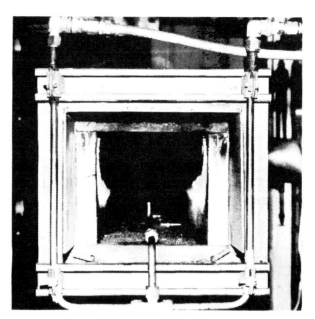

Figure 3. *Burner end of four-foot tunnel.*

deviation 1.5 inches) with red oak. These correspond to 25-foot tunnel flame-spread ratings of 0 and 100, respectively.

The asbestos-cement board reference material was fitted with thermocouples and radiometers to measure temperature and heat flux, respectively. The temperature was highest (above 900°C) about 8 inches from the fire end, and was below 500°C for most of the remainder of the tunnel length. Absorbed heat flux was generally less than 2 Btu per square foot per second.

TESTS ON MATERIALS

Twenty-five samples of rigid foams which had been previously tested in the 25-foot tunnel were tested in the laboratory tunnel. On the average, three specimens of each sample were tested under this standard set of operating conditions: air velocity 157.5 ft/min, heat supply rate 376 Btu/min, premixed air 56 percent. Test results are presented in Table 1, and the correlation obtained is presented in Figure 4.

The 25-foot tunnel flame spread ratings of 75 and 25 correspond to flame lengths of about 38 and 30 inches, respectively, in the 4-foot tunnel. For rough estimation, a flame length of 38 inches in the 4-foot tunnel would give a 50 percent chance of obtaining a 75 flame spread rating in the 25-foot tunnel, and a flame length of 30 inches would give a 50 percent chance of obtaining a 25 flame-spread rating.

One significant result of the initial work was a striking comparison between red oak and a commercial rigid foam with regard to reproducibility. While red oak, the

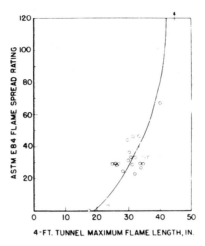

Figure 4. *Data obtained under less severe exposure conditions.*

recommended standard for ASTM E84, had a standard deviation of 1.5 inches (mean value 39.5 inches), Kode 25 had a standard deviation of 0.3 inch (mean value 28.3 inches).

Since it was highly desirable to develop predictive abilities in the 0 to 25 range of 25-foot tunnel flame-spread ratings, the standard operating conditions were adjusted to provide the greater exposure severity required. A large slab bun of Kode 25 was obtained so that this material could be used as the reference material for the high end of the desired range.

Relocation of the tunnel apparatus in another laboratory resulted in some changes in standard operating conditions. Reduction of propane supply pressure led to a decrease in the heat supply rate from 376 to 325 Btu per minute; this change, and changes in ductwork and laboratory configuration and conditions, required adjustment of the air supply rate to 240 feet per minute to give a flame length of 17.2 inches with asbestos-cement board. Under these conditions, the reference sample of Kode 25 gave a flame length of 30.0 inches.

Attempts to increase exposure severity by increasing air flow rate were not successful. Increasing air flow rate to 512 ft/min reduced the flame lengths with asbestos-cement board and Kode 25 to 16.2 inches and 17.7 inches, respectively, because of dilution with cold air and tilting of the flame away from the test surface. Exposure severity was finally increased by increasing the heat supply rate to 532 Btu per minute; the premixed air supplied to the burner was increased to about 66 percent of stoichiometric to provide a flame which the authors considered satisfactory in appearance. Air flow rate was maintained at 240 feet per minute. Under these conditions, asbestos-cement board gave a flame length of 21.5 inches (standard deviation 0.7 inch) and Kode 25 gave a flame length of 42.7 inches (standard deviation 0.6 inch). Materials intermediate between 0 and 25 flame spread were not available to the authors, because few if any rigid foams have flame spread ratings significantly lower than 25. A straight-line plot connecting the data points for asbestos-cement board and Kode 25 was selected because of this absence of intermediate data, and is shown in Figure 5. The authors estimate that a flame length of 43 inches under these more severe conditions would give a 50 percent chance of obtaining a 25 flame spread rating in the 25-foot tunnel.

To determine the sensitivity of test results to changes in heat supply rate, maximum flame lengths along asbestos-cement board and Kode 25 were measured at various levels of heat supply rate from 200 to 800 Btu per minute, maintaining

Table 1. Comparison of 25-Foot and 4-Foot Tunnel Test Results

Sample No.	ASTM E 84 Flame-Spread Rating	4-Foot Tunnel Maximum Flame Length, in.*
1	35.9	30.4 (1.8)
2	43.6	29.7 (1.7)
3	28.2	26.3 (1.8)
4	33.3	36.5 (5.5)
5	46.1	31.3 (4.1)
6	33.3	35
7	38.5	33.7 (3.8)
8	46.2	33.7 (5.2)
9	66.7	40
10	720	45.0 (3.0)
11	33.3	32.0 (4.2)
12	30.8	30.0
13	2.6	23.7 (0.3)
14	33.3	30.7 (4.4)
15	29.5	25.0 (1.2)
16	28.2	26.5 (0.6)
17	28.2	27.0 (2.0)
18	29.5	26.0 (1.0)
19	26.9	34
20	28.2	31.0 (8.0)
21	29.5	34.0 (7.0)
22	29.5	34.5 (5.5)
23	28.2	27.0 (1.2)
24	23.1	32.0 (4.0)
25 (Kode 25)	24.4	28.3 (0.3)
Asbestos-cement board	0	17.9 (0.7)
Red Oak	100	39.5 (1.5)

*Figures in parentheses are standard deviations.

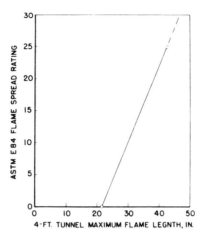

Figure 5. *Data obtained under more severe exposure conditions.*

premix air at 66 percent of stoichiometric and air flow rate at 240 feet per minute. Test results are presented in Figure 6. The asbestos-cement board became insensitive to increased heat supply above 500 Btu per minute, but the Kode 25 gave an essentially straight-line relationship over the 200-800 Btu per minute range.

All tests were conducted for a ten-minute period. The asbestos-cement board generally gave the same flame length over the entire ten-minute run, with the maximum observed flame length tending to occur during the last five minutes. With Kode 25, the maximum flame length was generally observed within the first minute. The

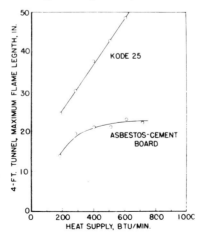

Figure 6. *Effect of heat flux on surface flame spread.*

111

use of Kode 25 as the reference material permits a much shorter test for control purposes, but at the same time requires more alertness on the part of the operator.

The straight-line relationship between maximum flame length observed with Kode 25 and the applied heat flux suggests that flame spread under forced convection along the surface of a self-extinguishing combustible material may be a linear function of the heat flux applied at the point from which flame spread is measured. Published work on flame spread over the surface of condensed-phase materials (14, 15, 16) has been concentrated on fuel beds consisting of combustible materials which were not self-extinguishing once the applied ignition source was removed. The authors are not aware of similar work on self-extinguishing combustible materials such as Kode 25.

CONCLUSIONS

The four-foot tunnel offers a means for predicting the results which might be obtained in the ASTM E 84 25-foot tunnel, and thereby permits screening of rigid foam candidates with substantial reductions in cost of sample preparation and testing.

Because of the sensitivity of test operation to external factors, each apparatus should be calibrated, using reference materials with known ratings.

The use of a self-extinguishing combustible material such as Kode 25 rigid foam as a reference material provides improved discrimination in the 25 flame-spread region. Flame spread along the surface of this material seems to be a linear function of the heat flux applied.

ACKNOWLEDGMENT

The Kode 25 reference material was supplied by Mr. H. G. Nadeau of the Upjohn Company and Mr. G. F. Bir of CPR Industries.

REFERENCES

1. A. J. Steiner, Underwriters' Lab. Res. Bull. No. 32 (September 1944).
2. Am. Soc. Testing Materials, ASTM E 84-70, ASTM Std. *14*, 395-403 (November 1971).
3. Underwriters' Laboratories, Std. UL 723 (March 1965).
4. National Fire Protection Assoc., Nat. Fire Codes *4*, 255-1 (1965).
5. C. C. Peters, and H. W. Eickner ASTM Spec. Tech. Publ. No. 344, 18-32 (October 1962).
6. Am. Soc. Testing Materials, ASTM E 286-69, ASTM Std. *14*, 508-513 (November 1971).
7. A. F. Robertson, D. Gross and J. J. Loftus, ASTM Proceedings *56*, 1437-1453 (1956).
8. Am. Soc. Testing Materials, ASTM E 162-67, ASTM Std. *14*, 480-490 (November 1971).
9. H. L. Vandersall, J. Paint Technology *39*, No. 511, 494-500 (August 1967).
10. M. M. Levy, Fire Technology *3*, No. 1, 38-46 (February 1967).
11. O. A. Krueger, K. C. Lyle and D. E. Jackson, J. Cellular Plastics *3*, No. 11, 497-501 (November 1967).
12. C. J. Hilado, "Flammability Handbook for Plastics," 48, Technomic Publishing Company, Westport, Connecticut (1969).
13. J. M. Kuchta, A. L. Furno and G. H. Martindill, Fire Technology *5*, No. 3, 203-216 (August 1969).

14. R. F. McAlevy, and R. S. Magee, "The Mechanism of Flame Spreading over the Surface of Igniting Condensed-Phase Materials," 12th International Symposium on Combustion Institute, Pittsburgh (1969).
15. C. Sanchez Tarifa, P. Perez del Notario, and P. Munoz Torralbo, "On the Process of Flame Spreading over the Surface of Plastic Fuels in an Oxidizing Atmosphere," 12th International Symposium on Combustion, 229-240, The Combustion Institute, Pittsburgh (1969).
16. J. N. de Ris, "Spread of a Laminar Diffusion Flame," 12th International Symposium on Combustion, 241-252, The Combustion Institute, Pittsburgh (1969).

Carlos J. Hilado

Carlos J. Hilado is a Project Scientist in the Fire Research Group of the Chemicals and Plastics Research and Development Department of Union Carbide Corporation at South Charleston, West Virginia. He received his B.S. degree in Chemical Engineering from De La Salle College in 1954 and his M.S. degree in Chemical Engineering Practice from Massachusetts Institute of Technology in 1956. He has been with Union Carbide Corporation since 1956 and has experience in vinyl and urethane foams, vinyl polymerization, testing and evaluation, industrial insulation, and flammability research.

Paul E. Burgess, Jr.

Paul E. Burgess, Jr. is Senior Research Chemist of Panacon Corporation at Cincinnati, Ohio. He received his B.S. degree in Mathematics in 1956 and his B.S. degree in Chemistry in 1957, both from Morris Harvey College. He served three years with the U.S. Air Force Weather Service, then worked with Union Carbide Corporation at South Charleston, West Virginia until 1971, when he joined Panacon Corporation. He has experience in the synthesis of organophosphorus and organoboron compounds, and the development of flame retardant rigid urethane foams.

C. P. BUTLER
Visiting Scientist

Northern Forest Fire Laboratory
Stanford Research Institute
Menlo Park, California

A SCHLIEREN SYSTEM FOR FIRE SPREAD STUDIES

(Received June 18, 1973)

ABSTRACT: A Schlieren optical system was devised for the purpose of studying free-flow fields of heated air above a fuel bed of pine needles ahead of an advancing fire.

Photographs were made at each of several distances from the flame front as it moved toward the center of the optical axis. Simultaneously, temperature measurements were made of a single exposed pine needle, representing a typical fuel element, located in the center of the fuel bed.

Selected pictures were analyzed to determine the flow field of the air above the fuel bed. The same photographs were used to establish a Schlieren temperature scale by visually comparing the optical contrast of the shadows with the actual temperature of the fuel particle.

INTRODUCTION

THE HEATING OF natural fuel elements on the ground ahead of an advancing fire is one factor in determining the rate of spread. Temperatures of pine needles exposed to an advancing flame front have been measured by Rothermel [1]. In the absence of wind, this heating is solely by radiation from the flame itself except at close distances when there may also be radiation from glowing embers.

The rising column of heated air above the fuel bed apparently lowers the pressure sufficiently so that the air along the ground ahead of the fire flows inward toward the fire. This flow field draws in ambient air which in turn convectively cools each exposed fuel element. Flame irradiance heats the side of the fuel element facing the fire while, at the same time, air flowing in the same direction cools the particle on the other side. The temperature of this particle at any time is therefore dependent on its optical and thermal properties as well as its dimensions and orientation. Its temperature, however, uniquely determines a convective transfer to the parcel of air immediately surrounding it, thus generating a rising column of air for each exposed particle. These columns, differing slightly in temperature from the air surrounding them, lend themselves to an analysis by Schlieren photography.

This type of photography employs an optical system made sensitive to slight changes in the index of refraction. Since the index of refraction for air changes with temperature, modestly heated parcels of air above the fuel bed can be readily photographed.

114

Columns of heated air are not normally visible in the forest because the background is not uniform and is usually very dark. The familiar shimmering of air directly over a tall stack on the other hand is readily visible because of uniform sky background. The background of a Schlieren system is uniformly illuminated, so that the slightest change in direction of a ray of light is magnified and shows up on the negative.

During the period of preheating, each exposed element of fuel ahead of an advancing fire becomes in turn a source of heat to warm the air immediately surrounding it. This gives rise to wavelets, or streamers, flowing upward from each fuel particle. These streamers expand and flow with the prevailing flow field. Beginning with laminar flow, they soon become turbulent and cease to be identifiable as proceeding from a particular particle of fuel.

If the system covers the lower few inches above the fuel bed, then individual streamers can easily be traced to an individual fuel particle. If this fuel element is then instrumented for temperature, a means is provided for a "Schlieren temperature scale" based on the visual appearance of the heated streamers of air and the actual temperature of the fuel element responsible for a particular streamer. Such a scale can be practical only in terms of calibration with a given type of fuel, although there is no theoretical reason why a calibration curve could not be constructed, based on the change of index with temperature together with convective heat transfer calculations from the fuel element to the air surrounding it.

OBJECTIVES OF A SCHLIEREN SYSTEM

Schlieren methods have been employed for many years for the measurement of convective flow of heated gases. Determination of the shape and flow patterns of shock waves around leading edges of wings and nose cones for re-entry vehicles are studied by means of such systems. Many studies of flame shapes have likewise used Schlieren methods in analysis. It must be emphasized that most work with this type of optical device has utilized very carefully designed parts mounted on stable supports and supplied with adjustable mechanisms for the alignment of all components, as described by Vasil'ev [2].

The purpose of the present study was to assess such a system for the examination of the flow field above a heated fuel bed. The results may be used to indicate exposed fuel bed features that cannot now be seen. The equipment available for this study was not designed for this specific purpose, and only rudimentary supports were used, in contrast to the usual Schlieren system. One purpose was to evaluate the flexibility of nonstandard instruments in this type of work.

Specific objectives were two-fold:

1. To measure photographically the flow fields of ascending air streams above a fuel bed of pine needles exposed to the flame radiation of an advancing fire front.

2. To establish a Schlieren temperature scale based on the photographic contrast of the flow fields calibrated with measured fuel particle temperatures.

WORK PLAN

A Z-type Schlieren system, shown in plan view in Figure 1 was set up in the combustion room of the Northern Forest Fire Laboratory.

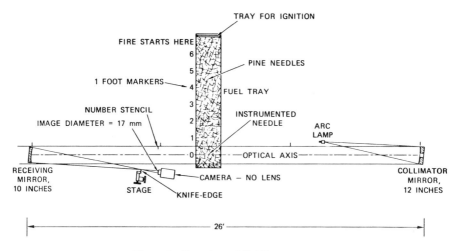

Figure 1. *Plan view of Schlieren system.*

The source of light was a 2-watt zirconium concentrated arc lamp, whose plasma filled an aperature 0.005 inch in diameter inside the lamp housing. This lamp makes an excellent approximation of a point source of light, rated by the manufacturer at 15,000 candles inch^2 [3].

The light from this lamp was collimated with a 12-inch-diameter, 72-inch-focal-length, front surface parabolic mirror. The mirror was provided with a 2-inch hole in the center for use in a Cassegrain telescope. At the receiving end of the optical system, the collimated beam was centered on a 10-inch-diameter, 83-inch-focal-length, front-surface parabolic mirror. Both mirrors were coated with aluminum.

At the focus of the second mirror, a knife edge, consisting of an ordinary razor blade was attached to a precision graduated mechanical stage. One motion was for focusing and the other for obscuring the image, i.e., for changing the sensitivity. If the image of the light source is completely cut off with the knife edge, then the only rays of light that will pass the edge will be those that have been bent through a large angle. We call this *dark field* illumination. However, if the knife edge is retracted until the whole image passes by, then the image on the photographic film is filled with light, which we designate as *bright field* illumination. At intermediate positions of the knife edge, the sensitivity can be varied at will to give a good contrast on the film.

Schlieren photographs were made at times when the flame front passed each of the 1-foot markers on the side of the fuel trays. Thus each photograph displays in the lower right-hand corner a number, corresponding to this distance.

Before each photograph was made, the knife edge was adjusted, as just described, to display the contrast of each flow field to the best advantage. This was a necessary part of each test, because of the instability of the supports, which often moved slightly due to uneven heating as the flame front approached. This knife edge adjustment to produce the maximum contrast for each setting would require monitoring if precise measurements were to be attempted.

Customarily, a Schlieren system (including both mirrors, knife edge supports and camera) is mounted on a rigid platform long enough to hold both ends of the optical system. This prevents relative motion between the source and the receiver ends, and assures that a given setting will remain constant. This refinement was not attempted here; instead all parts were screwed to plywood sheets resting on carpenter's saw horses. The knife-edge stage was held in place with laboratory clamps, rods, and a ring stand. While such an arrangement was awkward, and adjustments for high sensitivity could not be maintained for more than a few minutes, it was sufficient to make the tests.

Fuel trays in use at the laboratory measure 18 inches wide and 8 feet long, with a 3-inch-high supporting screen on either side to hold the fuel in a straight line. The tray was placed at right angles to the optical beam of the Schlieren system, so that a cylindrical volume of space directly above the fuel bed was sampled. This was located at one end, thus allowing measurements to be made of the heating by radiation to a distance of 7 feet from the flame front. The diameter of the sample volume was 10 inches and its length was approximately 18 inches. The beam traverses the full length, hence there may be several streamers of heated air in line with each other. In each photograph a few needles may be seen at the bottom, only one of which is instrumented with the thermocouple.

One needle in each test fire was split lengthwise and a 1-mil-diameter chromel-alumel thermocouple was inserted into the crack, which was then closed. The leads were carried out through the bottom of the fuel bed, and thence to a recording millivoltmeter, provided with temperature compensation, eliminating the need for a reference standard. The needle was carefully placed at the top of the fuel bed, centered in the middle of the optical system. A close up of one of these needles is shown in Figure 2.

The Schlieren photographs were made with a 35-mm motion picture camera equipped with a shutter that could be opened manually. The film takeup mechanism was powered with a hand-wound spring, and would expose 25 frames with one winding. No more than 2 or 3 frames were exposed at each distance of the flame from the center of the optical axis: rewinding was unnecessary for an entire run. Exposure time was set at 1/500 second for all exposures using black and white

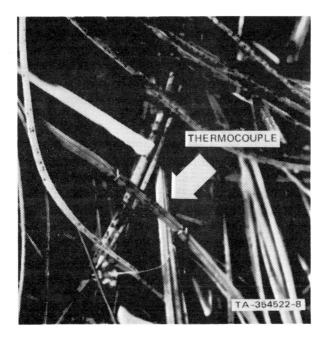

Figure 2. *Instrumented pine needle.*

Kodak Trix film. No lens was employed, so that scattered light in the room was bothersome until both the source and receiver ends were covered with black cloth, leaving only a small axial volume exposed along the optical axis. Some light was apparent during the time when the front edge of the flame was just coming into view at a distance of about 6 inches.

When the fuel tray had been loaded, weighed for the fuel loading, and pre-conditioned for several hours for moisture content, it was placed in position so that a few needles could be seen near the bottom of each photograph. The single instrumented needle was then carefully placed in the center of the bed and in line with the center of the optical system. This needle served as the fiducial point for the flame distance markers.

Ignition was accomplished by igniting 50 cc of acetone placed in a little metal trough at the opposite end of the bed from the Schlieren system. Shortly after ignition, the knife edge was adjusted and the first picture made when the distance from the needle to the flame front was 7 feet. At this time, the flame had reached its normal height of about 5 feet. In all photographs, the flame approaches from the right — i.e., from the same side as the distance number on each exposure. Sub-sequent exposures were made as the distance was reduced progressively. Simul-taneously with each exposure, the distance of the flame was recorded by marks on the thermocouple trace that recorded the temperature of the single needle.

EXPERIMENTAL RESULTS

Table 1 gives the fuel burning characteristics together with other parameters for analyzing fire spread in pine needles. The temperature rise of the pine needle tabulated here is shown graphically in Figure 3 as a function of the distance from the flame front. Schlieren photographs covering the same flame distances are shown in Figure 4 through 11.

Table 1. The Fuel and Its Burning Characteristics

Fuel type	Ponderosa pine needles
Fuel bed dimensions	18 in. by 8 ft
Fuel depth	3 in.
Fuel loading	0.50 lb/ft^2
Ambient air temperature	79° F
Relative humidity	23%
Average flame height (visually)	5 ft
Flame spread rate	0.75 ft/min.

Figure No.	Distance of Flame Front from Optical Axis (feet)	Pine Needle Temperature Rise above Ambient (°C)	Flow Field Direction, Degrees from Vertical (°)
4	7	0	—
5	6	3	—
6	5	6	60
7	4	8	70
8	3	10	45–55
9	2	17	55–65
10	1	33	50 90
11	0	175	40

Except for Figures 4 and 5 (the first two photographs) the direction of the flow field is clearly evident above the fuel bed. For Figures 6–11, the angle of the flow field is given in degrees measured from the vertical (see Table 1).

By the time the flame front is 1 foot away (Figure 10), it will be noted that the flow field bends a few inches above the top of the exposed needle and apparently flows horizontally directly into the base of the flame. At this distance, streamers from individual needles can be followed for at least 6 inches.

Figure 11 was taken when the flame front was just about even with the center of the field of view, perhaps a few inches beyond in some parts. The Schlieren patterns here are entirely different from any previous ones. The tiny star-shaped objects are flames, and may be small fireball bubbles. The temperature of the gases in these

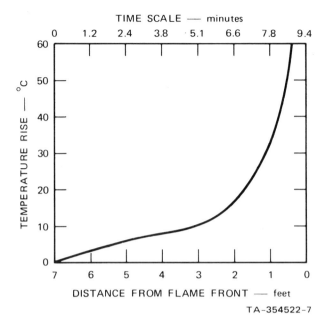

Figure 3. *Temperature rise of pine needle exposed to flame front.*

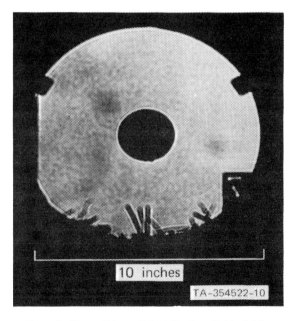

Figure 4. *Flame distance 7 feet. No flow fields visible.*
Temperature rise 0° C.

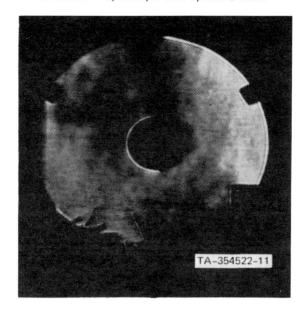

Figure 5. *Flame distance 6 feet. Flow fields visible, but appear random. Temperature rise $3°$ C.*

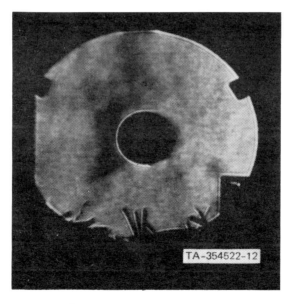

Figure 6. *Flame distance 5 feet. Flow field just visible ($60°$ from vertical). Temperature rise $6°$ C.*

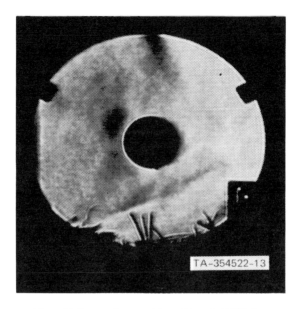

Figure 7. *Flame distance 4 feet. Flow field 70° from vertical. Temperature rise 8° C.*

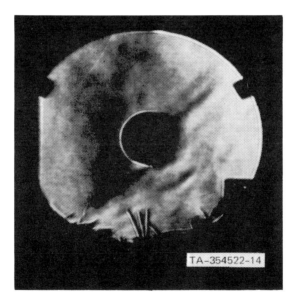

Figure 8. *Flame distance 3 feet. Flow field varies from 45° to 55° from vertical. Temperature rise 10°.*

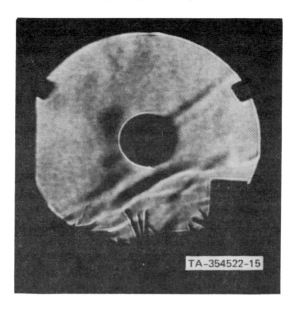

Figure 9. *Flame distance 2 feet. Flow field 55°–65° from vertical. Temperature rise 17° C (note increasing contrast of streamers).*

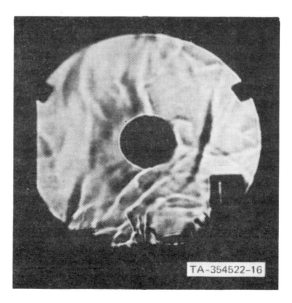

Figure 10. *Flame distance 1 foot. Flow field shows bending of streamers a few inches above fuel bed directly into base of flame to the right (50°–90°). Temperature rise 58° C (diameter of streamers is smaller than in previous figure and optical contrast is greater).*

123

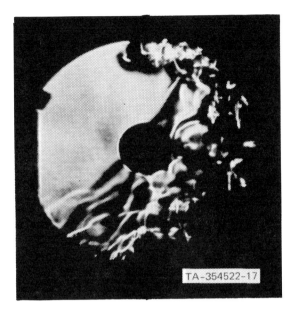

Figure 11. *Flame front is centered along optical axis giving distance of zero feet. Flow field just above and about 6 inches ahead of the flame appears to be undisturbed. Main flow is 40° from vertical. Stars may be fireball bubbles; at this knife-edge setting, light rays are bent beyond edge of mirror. Temperature is off scale.*

bubbles is very high, as may be judged by deflections of light extending beyond the edge of the mirror. Little can be said about the temperature of the pine needle at this time, because the temperature goes off scale rapidly as soon as the needle begins to burn.

A further significant feature of the last photograph is the volume of undisturbed air just in front of the flame. There is no apparent flow field in this region due to temperature gradients, even though the region is close to the flame front. This suggests that the air velocity in this region is flowing upward very fast, drawing in undisturbed ambient air.

It may be of interest to note the lowest temperature difference between the pine needle and the ambient air above it for which a Schlieren image with a barely discernible flow field can be recognized. Figure 5 shows a distinct pattern or disturbance extending up to about 10 inches above the fuel bed, although it is impossible to determine the direction of the flow field. This photograph corresponds to a temperature rise of 3°C, which, for the system used here may be considered the minimum temperature resolution. Temperature gradients of individual gas columns must be very low, yet the change in index is sufficient to reveal their outline, even at a distance of approximately 10 inches above the fuel bed.

Starting with Figure 5, a visual comparison of each photograph with the corresponding temperature rise of the pine needle provides a Schlieren temperature scale. With many more pictures than shown here, a scale could be made for which the temperature of the fuel particles could be read directly from the photographic images of the flow fields. Such a scale would be appropriate for any fuel similar to pine needles for example, excelsior.

CONCLUSIONS

The Schlieren system described provides a convenient method for studying the direction of the flow field above a heated fuel bed.

When correlated with the measured temperature of a pine needle exposed to the radiation of an advancing flame front, Schlieren images of the flow field produced by the heated fuel particle provides the basic data for a "Schlieren temperature scale."

REFERENCES

1. R. C. Rothermel, "A Mathematical Model for Predicting Fire Spread in Wildland Fuels," USDA Forest Service Paper INT-115 40 p. (1972).
2. L. A. Vasil'ev, "Schlieren Methods," translated by A. Baruch, Israel Program for Scientific Translation Keter, Inc., New York, Jerusalem, London (1971), xiv, 367 p.
3. Edmund Scientific Co., Catalog No. 731, p. 140.

Patrick J. Pagni

University of California
Berkeley, California 94720

QUANTITATIVE ANALYSIS OF PRESCRIBED BURNING

(Received May 15, 1972)

ABSTRACT: This paper is a compendium of two studies concerning a) measurements of fuel properties, flame characteristics and weather conditions at three range-improvement prescribed burns and b) an analytical model for steady state flame propagation through a thermally thin, porous fuel bed. The aim of this work is to quantitatively describe flame spread in prescribed burns so that fire behavior may be accurately predicted. Measurements are reported for the following fuel and terrain parameters: fuel loading, density, size, surface to volume ratio, moisture content, ground slope, air temperature, humidity, and wind velocity. Flame propagation rate, geometry, height and temperature are also included. The burned area is reexamined after the fire. In addition, an analysis of flame spread under conditions applicable to prescribed burns is summarized. The rate of energy transfer from the combustion zone to the fuel is assumed to control the rate of flame propagation. Energy transfer mechanisms considered are: flame and ember radiation, surface and internal convection, turbulent diffusion of flame eddies, and gas phase conduction. The effects of ambient flow, fuel moisture, fuel bed slope and endothermic porolysis are included. A nondimensional flame spread velocity is obtained as a function of nondimensional fuel, flame and ambient flow properties. Excellent agreement is obtained between model predictions and both field and laboratory data. It is hoped that this quantitative prediction of fire behavior will permit accurate use of prescribed burning in forest and range management.

I. INTRODUCTION

THE PROBLEM CONSIDERED is the quantitative description of flame spread under prescribed burn field conditions. Prescribed burning may be defined as the controlled use of fire at carefully selected times and locations to eliminate hazardous accumulated fuel. While this technique has been practiced for over thirty years, there exists no quantitative analysis for predicting the rates of spread and intensities of such fires. This lack of analytical understanding has logically led to a lack of confidence in this potentially useful fire prevention method. There exists, however, a critical need at this time to reduce fuel accumulation in our forests and grasslands.

Frequent low-intensity surface fires kept the primeval forest free of debris and understory trees and prevented high-intensity crown fires by reducing ground fuel accumulation [1]. Prescribed burning simulates this "ecological" fire control method. At a time of the year when the wildfire danger is minimal, a prescribed fire is ignited and allowed to propagate safely through the ground fuel layer. Since wildfires are often carried by this fuel, a successful prescribed burn will significantly reduce runaway wildfires during the peak fire season. However, if the safety and effectiveness of a prescribed burn are to be guaranteed, accurate prediction of the behavior of that fire is required. This provides the motivation for the attempt to predict flame spread rates and intensities for any given vegetative, topographical and meteorological conditions. The field measurements described here were performed during a National Science Foundation-Student Originated Studies project in the summer of 1971 [2]. While it is tempting to include the pedagogical details of that study, let it suffice to give credit to the members of the project for the data discussed here.

II. FIELD MEASUREMENTS OF FUEL AND FLAME CHARACTERISTICS

The problem considered in this section is determining what to measure at a prescribed burn and how to measure it to obtain experimental results which can serve as a basis for flame spread analysis. It was more convenient to instrument small field plots at prescribed burns which had been previously planned for range improvement, than to conduct experiments on laboratory fuel beds. This data supplements laboratory data available in the literature [3]. Much simplification is required before the methods described here can be adopted as a standard field procedure [4] for making burn — no burn decisions.

Measurements were made of the following fuel, topographic and weather parameters:

a)   Fuel size distribution, moisture content and density.
b)   Fuel surface to volume ratio and fuel bed depth and compactness.
c)   Preburn and postburn fuel distribution and loading.
d)   Topographic slope, wind speed and direction.
e)   Air temperature, humidity and pressure.

The following flame properties were also measured:

a)   Flame spread rate.
b)   Flame height, depth and angle.
c)   Time-temperature curves.

A field measurement heuristic was developed which included: sampling methods for vegetation characterization, a size class determiner, an abney for slope measurement, an anemometer to obtain wind speed and direction and a sling psychrometer for air temperature and humidity. Photographic techniques were used for flame length, depth, and rate of propagation, and shielded thermocouples and fusible temperature indicators supplied temperature data. In the laboratory, toluene distillation gave moisture content data, while water immersion of saturated samples gave fuel density data. Mineral content analysis was supplied by a professional laboratory.

127

For sampling in woodland and grassland areas, stratified random sampling [5] with one meter square quadrats as sampling units was found most useful. The fuels found in these quadrats were divided into size classes from which their fuel characteristics were later determined. Sampling in chaparral-type areas called for the line-transect method of sampling [5]. In this technique, lengths of ten meter string were randomly placed and the various species crossing the string were recorded. Both sampling methods yielded satisfactory results. It was found that the main problems encountered in sampling fuel characteristics were not of a statistical nature but rather involved the mechanics of obtaining unaltered samples. For a more detailed discussion of sampling methods see Reference 1.

In the summer of 1971 three prescribed burns were instrumented on ranches in San Benito, Napa and Mariposa Counties within 150 miles of Berkeley. On each ranch a sample plot 40 by 20 meters was isolated from the prescribed burn area by a bulldozed fuel break and instrumented as shown in Figure 1. The plots were chosen to have homogeneous fuel loading with the fire propagating uphill in the direction of the prevailing wind. The plot was uniformly ignited along the windward short side. Photographic stations, indicated by R1, ... R5 and L1, ... L5 were marked along the side of the plot to record flame characteristics. Weather monitoring equipment and tape recorders were carried in the fuel break next to the flame. Eight instrument stations were located in the plot as indicated in Figure 1.

Figure 2 is a side view of the Wilbur Ranch plot showing two of these instrument stations. A curved flame front is propagating through high grass from right to left. An instrument station schematic, with shielded thermocouples shown in detail, is given in Figure 3. Time-temperature histories in a matrix of four vertical positions at three locations could be obtained using a strip chart recorder with a portable power source. Tempilstiks ® were also used to obtain maximum temperature as a function of height at each station.

In preliminary studies such as this, photographic data provide useful information as shown in Figures 4 and 5. Both standard and infrared film were used at the Guenoc Ranch to record flame characteristics. Figure 4a is a visible light photograph of a flame propagating through *Adenostoma* sp. (greasewood) while 4b shows the same location and time photographed using 35 mm infrared film with a sensitivity cutoff at .9 microns. Comparison of Figures 4a and 4b indicates that the sources of the visible and the detected infrared radiation are nearly identical; thus visible flame characteristics may suffice for approximate heat transfer calculations.

The ability of a prescribed burn to reduce hazardous accumulated fuel is well illustrated by Figures 5a and 5b. The fuel on the Guenoc Ranch was uniform greasewood brush providing quite a different set of fuel parameters from those encountered with the grassy fuel on the Wilbur Ranch. Figure 5a shows the preburn fuel loading and relative size; Figure 5b shows postburn fuel loading at the same location. Note that primarily the finer fuel is burned. The overall fuel reduction was ~ 60% by weight while fuel with a diameter greater than 2 cm was reduced by less than 7% and fuel with a diameter less than .5 cm was completely eliminated. This

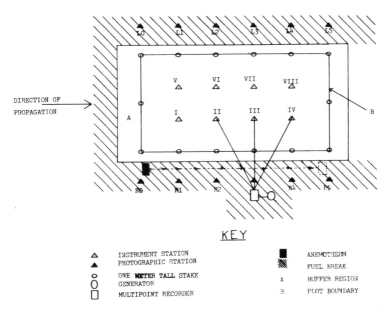

KEY

△	INSTRUMENT STATION	■	ANEMOTHERM
▲	PHOTOGRAPHIC STATION	▨	FUEL BREAK
○	ONE METER TALL STAKE	A	BUFFER REGION
○	GENERATOR		
▢	MULTIPOINT RECORDER	B	PLOT BOUNDARY

Figure 1. *Prescribed burn sample plot geometry and instrumentation plan.*

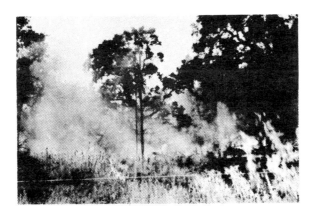

Figure 2. *Photograph of a typical prescribed
burn with instrument station in center (Wilbur Ranch).*

129

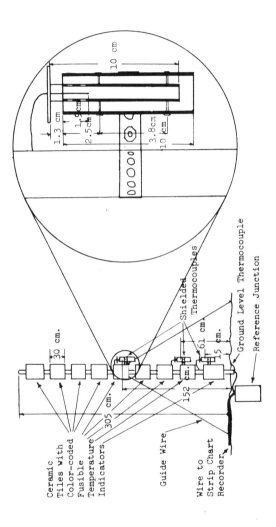

Figure 3. *Instrument station schematic showing shielded thermo-couples and fusible temperature indicators.*

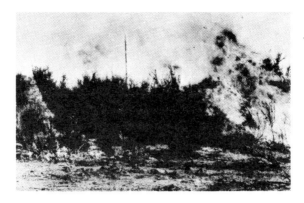

Figure 4a. *Photograph of flame propagating through Adeno-stoma sp. on Guenoc Ranch, Middletown, California, August 22, 1971.*

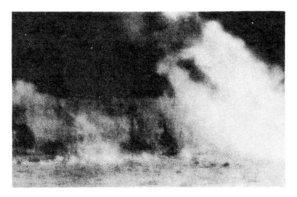

Figure 4b. *Infrared photograph taken at the same time and location as Figure 4a.*

indicates that only the fine fuel is involved in the initial propagation of the flame and only this fuel should be incorporated in analytical propagation models.

The most complete data were obtained at the third prescribed burn. Only these data are reported here. At the Wilbur and Guenoc Ranches the fuel distribution was relatively uniform; however, at the Long Ranch, it was quite heterogeneous. Preburn and postburn maps showing the location and size of the various generic types of fuel in the Long Ranch sample plot are given by Figures 6a and 6b. The fraction of the plot occupied by each type of vegetation can be estimated from Figure 6a to permit calculation of mean fuel characteristics if desired. Postburn examination correlated qualitative information from previous fires that tar weed (*Hemizonia* sp.) would not ignite. Preburn fuel sampling data, neglecting non-burning fuels, are given in Table 1. Approximate surface to volume ratios were developed for: a) cylinder like fuel: $S/V = 4/D$; b) flat fuel: $S/V = 2/\ell_t$; and c) pine

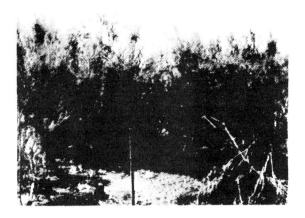

Figure 5a. *Photograph of preburn fuel loading in sample plot on the Guenoc Ranch.*

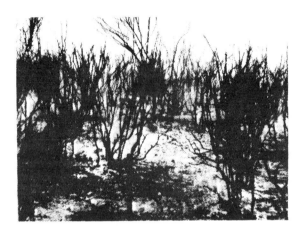

Figure 5b. *Photograph of postburn fuel loading at same location as Figure 5a.*

needles: $S/V = 2.5/\ell_t$, where D is the diameter and ℓ_t is the thinnest thickness. Results of these approximations for the Long Ranch fuel are given in column 4 of Table 1.

Mariposa County is particularly dry and hot in August and, thus, there was relatively little moisture in the fuel as shown in column 1 of Table 1. On the day of the burn the temperature was near 30°C with a relative humidity of less than 10%. The fuel depth of the grassy areas was 25 cm while the brush depth was 173 cm. The average fuel compactness was .13 cm^{-1}. These conditions combined with the relatively steep slope resulted in flame speeds an order of magnitude higher than the previous burns.

Intense heat from the flames on both sides of the lefthand fuel-break forced the

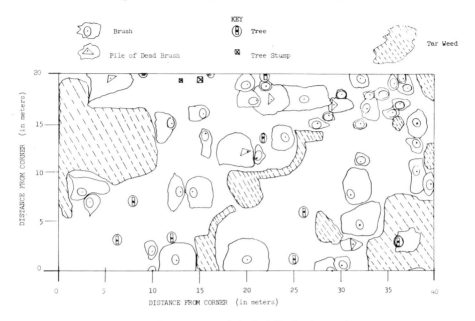

Figure 6a. *Preburn map of the fuel distribution on the
Long Ranch sample plot.*

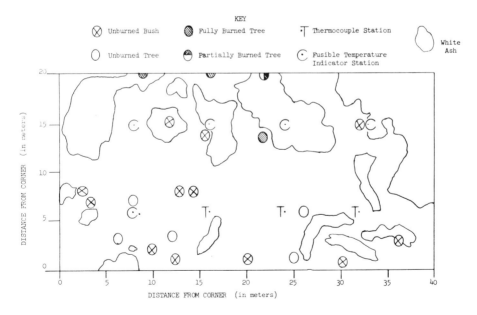

Figure 6b. *Postburn map of the Long Ranch sample plot (to be
compared with Figure 6a).*

133

Table 1. Average Preburn Fuel Properties for each Fuel Type on the
Long Ranch Sample Plot

Fuel Type (by size)	% Moisture Content (water mass/dry fuel mass) $\times 10^2$	Density $(gm\text{-}cm^{-3})$	Surface to Volume Ratio (cm^{-1})	Loading $(gm\text{-}cm^{-2})$
Ground cover (duff)	4.9	.63	105	221
Grass	3.5	.33	120	73
Small Brush	—	.28	13	45
Large Brush	6.2	.56	4	176
Lower Tree Branches	9.7	.61	19	—
Average Overall	5	.5	105	
Total				515

abandonment of photographic techniques on that side of the plot. All pictures taken in this fire were from Stations R1 through R4 (see Figure 1) as indicated in column 2 of Table 2. Column 1 of Table 2 gives the time from ignition. Columns 3 through 6 contain average flame characteristics obtained from visible light photographs. Flame length is defined as the maximum extension of the flame. This dimension coupled with the vertical flame height defines the flame tilt angle which is positive in the direction of propagation. Flame depth is the maximum horizontal dimension of the fire. The wind speed in meters per second (divide by 2.24 to obtain miles per hour) is listed in column 7. The wind direction was from the south, $\pm 45°$. The fire was moving toward the northeast up the slope indicated in column 8 of Table 2. Column 9 lists average flame spread rates in meters per second for sample plot segments of constant slope. Fahnestock's dichotomous key [4] predicted a spread rate of .037 m/sec for the sample plot. This key provides a useful tool for qualitatively evaluating fuel properties. However, the effects of wind and slope on flame characteristics must also be considered.

Figure 7 shows time-temperature histories measured by the shielded thermocouples at station IV (see Figure 1). The time from ignition of the plot is indicated on the abscissa. The fact that all thermocouples reached approximately the same maximum temperature would indicate that to the accuracy of the measurement the flame temperature was uniform with height. The data described here are only a rough beginning, but they provide valuable information for the formulation of an analytical model for flame spread.

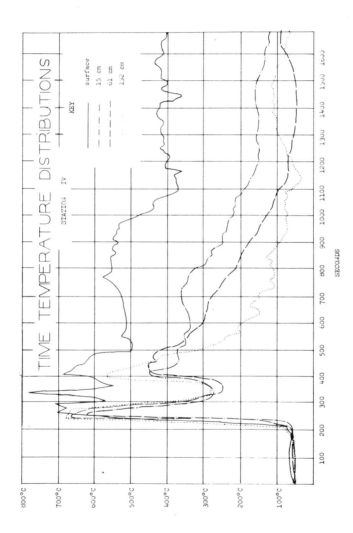

Figure 7. *Typical temperature histories as measured by the shielded thermocouples shown in Figure 3 (Long Ranch).*

Table 2. Flame Characteristics, Wind Speed, Ground Slope and Flame Spread Rate as a Function of Time on the Long Ranch Sample Plot

time (Min: sec)	station desig- nation	flame length (cm)	flame height (cm)	maximum flame depth (cm)	flame direc- tion	wind speed (m/sec)	slope (%)	rate of flame spread (m/sec)
0:14	RO	30	20	70	+	—	14	0.444
0:18	RO	120	100	200	+	2.49	14	0.444
0:21	RO	80	60	500	+	2.18	14	0.444
0:27	R1	25	20	5	+	1.57	16	0.661
0:42	R2	600	600	600		1.55	16	0.203
0:44	R2	600	600	600		1.60	16	0.203
0:50	R2	600	600	600		1.49	16	0.203
0:55	R3	550	400	350	+	1.36	19	0.060
1:18	R3	550	320	600	+	1.83	19	0.060
1:22	R3	—	—	250	+	1.90	19	0.060
1:27	R3	—	1000	—	+	1.98	19	0.060
2:11	R4	450	400	—	+	1.66	18	0.031
3:26	R4	—	180	—		1.89	18	0.031
4:09	R4	150	150	50	0	2.13	18	0.031
4:18	R4	—	150	150	+	1.56	18	0.031
4:39	R4	60	60	100	+	1.36	18	0.031
4:42	R4	200	200	350	+	1.69	18	0.031
4:47	R4	70	70	350	+	1.26	18	0.031

III. ANALYTICAL MODEL

Ideally, the prediction of fire behavior should be based only on preburn fuel, topography and weather measurements. The first step, however, is to correctly model the propagation of a given flame through a given fuel bed. Once the energy transfer mechanisms have been accurately quantified, the analysis can be extended to obtain flame properties. These properties are required a priori along with the fuel bed and ambient flow properties in the calculations reported here.

An analysis describing steady, quasi-one-dimensional flame propagation through a porous, fuel bed has been developed [6, 7]. It is assumed that the rate of flame spread is controlled by the rate of energy transfer from the flame to the fuel. Prescribed burning is well represented by including wind velocity, moisture content and slope in this simple model. The rate controlling energy transfer mechanisms include: radiation from flame and embers, convection above and through the fuel bed, and gas phase conduction. When this energy is absorbed at the fuel bed, moisture is evaporated, fuel is pyrolysed and unignited fuel is heated to an ignition condition.

The following assumptions are made to obtain a simple mathematical model for this complex physical process: 1) chemical kinetics is infinitely fast, therefore, the flame may be represented by a flame sheet; 2) the propagation process is steady, therefore a constant propagation velocity, R, exists; 3) the flow field is one-dimensional, i.e., the fuel and the gas are thermally thin; 4) ignition of the fuel bed occurs when the fuel reaches an ignition temperature; 5) solid phase conduction is initially neglected since the gas phase temperature gradients are an order of magnitude higher than the solid phase temperature gradients.

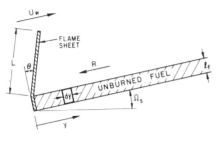

Figure 8. *Notation and physical model for the flame and fuel bed used to analytically determine the flame spread rate.*

As shown in Figure 8, in the reference frame of the flame, the fuel bed moves into the flame sheet with the flame speed, R. The flame length is L and the angle between the flame sheet and the normal to the fuel bed is θ. The ambient flow velocity relative to the fuel in the direction of flame propagation is U_w. The thickness of the actually burned fuel bed is ℓ_f. The slope angle is Ω_s. The origin is placed at the end of the fuel bed next to the flame. Gas phase conduction is included by displacing the flame a distance, $-\delta$, a fuel diffusion length, from the fuel bed.

Consider an elemental control volume of width dy and height ℓ_f in the fuel bed a distance y ahead of the flame as indicated in Figures 8 and 9. Energy conservation may be written

$$\text{Ignition Energy} = \text{Adsorbed Preheating Energy} \tag{1}$$

$$
\left.\begin{array}{l}
q_s\text{(sensible energy)} \\[4pt]
+\, q_v\text{(moisture)} \\[4pt]
+\, q_p\text{(pyrolysis)}
\end{array}\right\}
=
\left\{\begin{array}{l}
q_{rf}\text{(flame radiation)} + q_{rb}\text{(ember radiation)} \\[4pt]
+\, q_{cs}\text{(surface convection)} + q_{ci}\text{(interior convection)} \\[4pt]
+\, q_{kg}\text{(gas conduction)} + q_{ct}\text{(turbulent diffusion)}
\end{array}\right.
$$

Starting at the left hand side, the terms in Equation 1 represent: the increase in fuel sensible energy, the moisture evaporation energy, an endothermic energy of pyrolysis, radiant heating from the flame, radiant heating from the embers, convective heating of the fuel bed surface, convective heating within the fuel bed, gas phase conduction and convective heating due to turbulent flame eddies. A detailed derivation of each term in Equation 1 as a function of flame, fuel and ambient properties is available [6, 7]. The integral of Equation 1 from ambient conditions (y = ∞) to the flame (y = 0) equates the total energy required to ignite a fuel element to the total energy received during preheating.

The resulting nondimensional flame propagation rate, Π_V, is obtained as a function of nondimensional energy transfer parameters as

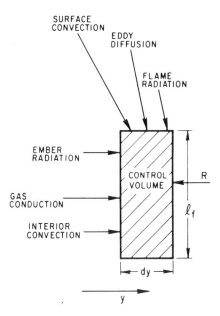

Figure 9. *Fuel bed control volume with preheating energy transfer mechanisms indicated.*

$$\Pi_V = \frac{\Pi_C[\Pi_{CT} + \Pi_W\Pi_{CI} + \Pi_W^{4/5}\Pi_{CS}] + (\Pi_{RF} + \Pi_{RB}) + \Pi_K}{(1 + \Pi_M + \Pi_{PYR})} \qquad (2)$$

with

$$\Pi_V = \frac{R\phi\rho_f c_{pf}(T_{ig}-T_\infty)}{E_{f\ell}} \,, \quad \Pi_M = \frac{M_{w\infty}h_{vap}}{c_{pf}(T_{ig}-T_\infty)} \,, \quad \Pi_{PYR} = \frac{M_{pf}h_{pyr}}{c_{pf}(T_{ig}-T_\infty)} \,,$$

$$\Pi_C = \frac{c_{pg}\rho_g(T_{f\ell}-T_f)\sqrt{gL}}{E_{f\ell}} \,, \Pi_{CS} = \frac{.2(L)^{4/5}\nu_g^{1/5}}{\ell_f(gL)^{1/10}} \,, \quad \Pi_{CT} = \frac{k_c}{\ell_f\sqrt{gL}}$$

$$\Pi_{CI} = \frac{1}{1 + \dfrac{7.5\ell_c N_c \nu_g^{4/3} D_c^{2/3}}{\Pi_W^{1/3}s\,\alpha_g(gL)^{1/6}}} \,, \quad \Pi_W = \frac{U_w}{\sqrt{gL}} \,, \quad \Pi_{RF} = \frac{a}{2}\left(\frac{L}{\ell_f}\right)(1 + \sin\theta).$$

$\Pi_{RB} = E_b/E_{f\ell}$, $\Pi_K = k_g(T_{f\ell}-T_{ig})/\delta_g E_{f\ell}$ and $\theta = \Omega_s + \tan^{-1}(1.4\,\Pi_W)$ where Π_V is the ratio of the actual flame velocity to the velocity due to radiation alone; Π_M is the ratio of the evaporation enthalpy to the fuel energy increase required for ignition; Π_{PYR} is the ratio of the pyrolysis enthalpy to the fuel energy increase; Π_C

is the ratio of the buoyant energy flux to the radiation energy flux; Π_K is the ratio of the conduction energy flux to the radiation energy flux; Π_{CT}, Π_{CI} and Π_{CS} measure the turbulent diffusion, the internal convection and the surface convection, respectively; Π_{RF} describes the geometric dependence of the flame radiation flux; Π_{RB} is the ratio of the ember radiation to the flame radiation and Π_W is the ratio of the wind speed to the buoyant velocity. Other notation is defined in the nomenclature list. The solution details [6, 7] are omitted here.

When no ambient flow exists, $\Pi_W = 0$, and the flame-tilt angle is the slope angle, $\theta = \Omega_S$. For a flame propagating into the ambient flow, there is neither surface nor internal convective heating; thus, $\Pi_C \Pi_W \Pi_{CI}$ and $\Pi_C \Pi_W^{4/5} \Pi_{CS}$ are identically zero. For the case of $\ell_f \approx L$ and very porous fuel, e.g., grass, surface convection is neglected. Similarly for fuel beds which are extremely porous, e.g., pine needle beds, internal convection is neglected.

Figure 10 shows the dependence of the nondimensional flame speed, Π_V, on the nondimensional ambient wind speed, Π_W, parameterized in a nondimensional moisture evaporation energy, Π_M, as given in Equation 2. The nondimensional pyrolysis energy, Π_{PYR}, convected energy, Π_C, conducted energy, Π_K, and radiated energies, Π_{RF} and Π_{RB}, were held fixed at mean values for the Long Ranch plot [2] shown in Figure 10. The exponential increase of Π_V displays the exponential dependence of the flame radiation to the fuel bed on the ambient velocity, Π_W.

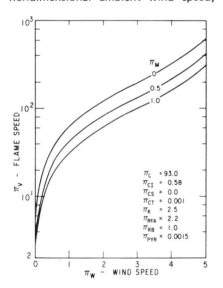

Figure 11 gives a comparison of the predicted and experimental nondimensional flame speeds for the data obtained at the prescribed burns described in Section II. Good quantitative agreement is indicated. The 45° line is the locus of exact agreement. This method of cross-plotting the predicted and experimental results is necessitated by the fact that each experimental point has an entirely different set of nondimensional energy transfer parameters; therefore, no common set exists, as in Figure 10. A wide variety of fuel, flame and ambient parameters is represented. Since all fuel beds were very porous — grass at the Wilbur Ranch, brush at the Guenoc Ranch and grass and brush at the Long Ranch, internal convection dominates and the surface convection, Π_{CS}, was taken as zero.

Figure 10. *Nondimensional flame speed, Π_V, versus nondimensional wind speed, Π_W, parameterized in nondimensional moisture content, Π_M, for flame and fuel parameters typical [2] of brush and grass on the Long Ranch sample plot.*

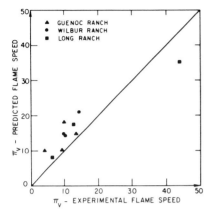

Figure 11. *Comparison of predicted and experimental nondimensional flame speeds for three instrumented prescribed burns. The 45° line is the exact agreement locus. Good quantitative agreement is indicated.*

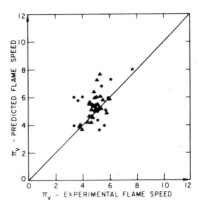

Figure 12. *Comparison of predicted and experimental nondimensional flame speeds for white pine needle ● and ponderosa pine needle ▲ laboratory fires with no wind. The 45° line is the exact agreement locus. Good quantitative agreement is indicated.*

Prescribed burning is also utilized in the opposite extreme of only slightly porous fuel, such as pine needle beds. A comparison with laboratory data [3] obtained with no ambient flow in white and ponderosa pine needle fuel beds is shown in Figure 12. Good agreement is illustrated for both species. Additional comparisons are available [6, 7].

IV. CONCLUDING REMARKS

It is hoped that the methodologies developed here will prove useful. These data supplement and support measurements on man-made fuel beds [3]. It remains to develop a routine sampling system for use prior to prescribed burns to determine whether optimum burning conditions exist. Simple dichotomous keys [4] may be quite useful, since the engineering properties of vegetation show small variation; however, ambient flow properties and topography must be included. Perhaps this can be accomplished using small computers, centrally located and equipped with a visual CRT display of a fire's predicted progress.

A flame spread model, incorporating wind and slope effects, which describes steady, quasi-one dimensional flame propagation through a thermally-thin, porous fuel bed has been applied to flame spread in prescribed burns. The model predictions are in good quantitative agreement with field and laboratory data. Flame spread rates under prescribed burning conditions are predictable if flame characteristics (height and intensity) as well as fuel bed parameters are known. The agreement between experimental and predicted flame spread rates verifies that the heat transfer mechanisms are correctly modeled. However, complete prediction of fire behavior under prescribed burn conditions requires prediction of all flame characteristics (spread rate, height, intensity, and fuel reduction) using only pre-burn fuel bed parameter measurements as input. The complete analysis consists of the following steps:

1) Approximate pyrolysis rates and product species are defined as functions of temperature.
2) A fuel bed temperature distribution is assumed.
3) Approximate flame temperatures are calculated assuming rich combustion of gaseous fuel at a rate consistent with step 1.
4) Energy released by the flame is calculated using the flame temperature obtained in step 3 with a fluid mechanic model for the flame height and geometry.
5) The energy input to the fuel bed, the flame spread rate and the temperature distribution in the fuel bed are calculated using the model described here.
6) The assumed temperature distribution in step 2 is replaced with the temperature distribution derived in step 5, and steps 2 through 6 are iterated until flame characteristics converge.

This quantitative model of flame characteristics under prescribed burning conditions is not trivial, but it can be readily accomplished.

V. ACKNOWLEDGMENTS

The author gratefully acknowledges the assistance of T. Peterson, L. Houck, D. Pearl, R. Buckius, A. Carlson, F. Dodd, W. Garetz, D. Cherkin, D. Kelley, J. Boyd, S. Boghosian, D. Ng, Q. Kwan, R. Pendleton and S. Gish.

Special thanks are extended to the staff and owners of the Wilbur, Guenoc and Long Ranches. The aid of the Pacific Southwest Forest and Range Experiment Station of the U.S. Forest Service, the School of Forestry and Conservation, University of California, Berkeley, and the State Division of Forestry is greatly appreciated.

This research was sponsored by National Science Foundation Grants GY-9112 and GI-43.

REFERENCES

1. H. Biswell and H. Weaver, "Redwood Mountains," *American Forests, 74*; 8, 20-23, August 1968.
2. P. J. Pagni, L. D. Houck, T. G. Peterson, R. Pendleton, D. Pearl, D. Ng, Q. Kwan, D. Kelley, S. Gish, W. Garetz, F. Dodd, D. Cherkin, A. Carlson, R. Buckius, J. Boyd and S. Boghosian, "Prescribed Burning," Report No. TS-71-5, College of Engineering, University of California, Berkeley, December 1971.
3. R. C. Rothermal and H. E. Anderson, "Fire Spread Characteristics Determined in the Laboratory," U.S. Department of Agriculture, Forest Service Research Paper INT-30, 1966.
4. G. R. Fahnestock, "Two Keys for Appraising Forest Fire Fuels," U.S. Department of Agriculture, Forest Service Research Paper PNW-99, 1970.

5. P. Greig-Smith, *Quantitative Plant Ecology* (Academic Press, Inc., New York, 1957).
6. T. G. Peterson and P. J. Pagni, "Spread of a Preheating Flame Through Porous Fuel," College of Engineering Report No. TS-72-1, Mechanical Engineering Department, University of California, Berkeley, March 1972.
7. P. J. Pagni and T. G. Peterson, "Flame Spread Through Porous Fuels," to be presented at and published in the Proceedings of the Fourteenth Symposium (International) on Combustion, The Combustion Institute, August 1972.

NOMENCLATURE

a	fuel absorptivity
a_p	pre-exponential $[t^{-1}]$
c_p	specific heat $[EM^{-1}T^{-1}]$
D	mass diffusivity $[L^2 t^{-1}]$
D_c	average diameter of approximately cylindrical fuel particles [L]
D	eddy diffusivity $[L^2 t^{-1}]$
E	emissive power $[E\ L^{-2} t^{-1}]$
E_p	activation energy for pyrolysis $[EM^{-1}]$
h	heat transfer coefficient $[EL^{-2}T^{-1}t^{-1}]$
h_{pyr}	specific endothermic enthalpy of pyrolysis $[EM^{-1}]$
h_{vap}	heat of vaporization of water plus specific enthalpy required to reach $212°F$ $[EM^{-1}]$
k_c	proportionality constant for turbulent diffusion preheating O(1)
k	thermal conductivity $[EL^{-1}T^{-1}t^{-1}]$
L	flame length [L]
Le	Lewis number
ℓ_c	average length of approximately cylindrical fuel particles [L]
ℓ_f	thickness of fuel layer initially burned [L]
m_f'	mass flux of pyrolyzed volatiles $[ML^{-2}t]$
M_p	fraction of initial fuel mass that remains unpyrolyzed at y
M_w	moisture content (ratio of mass of water to mass of dry fuel at y)
N_c	average number of cylinders per unit volume of fuel bed, $[L^{-3}]$
Pr	Prandtl number
q	energy per unit fuel bed volume per unit time $[EL^{-2}t^{-1}]$
R	steady-state flame spread velocity $[Lt^{-1}]$
s	fuel surface area per unit volume of fuel bed $[L^{-1}]$
T	temperature [T]
U_w	ambient flow velocity $[Lt^{-1}]$
y	distance into fuel bed from flame [L]
α	thermal diffusivity $[L^2 t^{-1}]$
δ	flame standoff distance [L]
ϵ	emissivity
θ	angle between flame sheet and fuel bed normal
ν	kinematic viscosity $[L^2 t^{-1}]$

Π_C dimensionless convection coefficient
Π_{CI} dimensionless internal convection
Π_{CS} dimensionless surface convection
Π_{CT} dimensionless turbulent diffusion
Π_K dimensionless gas phase conduction
Π_M dimensionless evaporation enthalpy
Π_{PYR} dimensionless pyrolysis enthalpy
Π_{RB} dimensionless ember radiation
Π_{RF} dimensionless flame radiation
Π_V dimensionless flame velocity
Π_W dimensionless wind velocity
ρ density $[ML^{-3}]$
ϕ ratio of solid fuel volume to fuel bed volume
Ω_S slope angle of fuel bed
Ω_W tilt angle of flame due to the wind, $\tan^{-1}\left[\dfrac{1.4U_w}{(gL)^{1/2}}\right]$

Subscripts

b   ember
f   dry fuel
fℓ flame
g   gas
ig   ignition
O $y = O$ (at flame)
∞ $y = \infty$ (ambient condition)